MW01516945

Garibaldi Secondary School
24789 Dewdney Trunk Road
Maple Ridge, B.C.
V4R 1X2

Nutrition & You

Nutrition: A Global View

Books in This Series

Nutrition & Politics

Nutrition & Poverty

Nutrition & Science

Nutrition & Society

Nutrition & You

Garibaldi Secondary School
24789 Dewdney Trunk Road
Maple Ridge, B.C.
V4R 1X2

Nutrition
& You

Ida Walker

AlphaHouse Publishing
New York

Nutrition: A Global View
Nutrition & You

Copyright © 2009 by AlphaHouse Publishing, a division of PEMG Publishing Group. All rights reserved. No part of this publication may be reproduced or transmitted in any form or by any means, electronic or mechanical, including photocopying, recording, taping, or any information storage and retrieval system, without permission from the publisher.

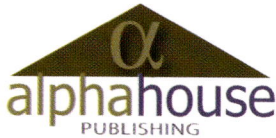

alphahouse
PUBLISHING

AlphaHouse Publishing
A Division of PEMG Publishing Group, Inc.
201 Harding Avenue
Vestal, New York 13850
www.alphahousepublishing.com

First Printing
9 8 7 6 5 4 3 2 1
ISBN: 978-1-934970-33-1
ISBN (set): 978-1-934970-28-7
    Library of Congress Control Number: 2008930659
Author: Walker, Ida

Cover design by Wendy Arakawa.
Interior design by MK Bassett-Harvey.

Printed in India by International Print-O-Pac Limited

An ISO 9001 Company

Contents

Introduction to Nutrition:

A Global View

Many young adults are used to looking at nutrition in the context of health classes and home economics classes. Most of them know that nutrition is a critical component for healthy development, one that is connected to energy levels, strong bones and teeth, clear skin, reduced risk for infectious diseases, and other physical outcomes. But students may be far less aware that nutrition also has global consequences. It is an issue that pertains to social studies, economics, current events, and science studies.

In our global world, nutrition issues have enormous importance. Food crises and world hunger are only the most visible and urgent tip of the malnourishment iceberg. Beneath the world's waters lurks an even more pervasive danger. At least one-fifth of the worldwide loss of years of life to death and to disability is due to hunger and undernutrition. If diet-related chronic diseases (such as diabetes, obesity, and hypertension) are taken into consideration, some experts believe that as much as one-half of the world's illnesses and mortality can be attributed to malnutrition.

As future citizens and leaders, young adults need to understand that investing in the world's nutrition is vital to the well-being of the global community. Improved nutrition empowers people and communities; it fuels the development process and leads to political, economic, and social renewal. Empowered and well-nourished communities are also less likely to be drawn into wars and violent conflicts. In an increasingly interconnected world, the payoff for global good nutrition is higher than ever.

The United Nations is well aware of this connection; the rights of all individuals to appropriate and adequate nutrition are embedded in six of the universal proclamations included in the 1990 World Declaration and Plan of Action on the Survival, Protection and Development of Children. Kofi Annan, former Secretary General of the United Nations, has written:

> The world knows what is needed to end malnutrition. With a strong foundation of cooperation between local communities, non-governmental organizations, governments, and international agencies, the future—and the lives of our children—can take the shape we want and they deserve, of healthy growth and development, greater productivity, social equity, and peace.

The books in this series, Nutrition: A Global View, will help students build the knowledge base and the perspectives necessary to help achieve these vital goals.

—*Dr. Peter Vash*

Here's what you need to know

- Good nutrition comes from the parts of food that help our bodies to do their jobs.
- Malnutrition means not getting enough of the foods you need to be healthy.
- The nutrients (the part of food that provides nutrition) that your body needs are calories, carbohydrates, fat, protein, vitamins, minerals, fiber, and water.
- A calorie is a way to measure how much energy a food offers your body.
- You need one gram (about a third of an ounce) of protein per kilogram of weight (0.4 grams per pound).
- Carbohydrates give you energy. If you eat too many carbohydrates, they will be converted into body fat.
- About 30 percent of your daily calories should come from fat in order for your body to be healthy.
- You need smaller amounts of vitamins and minerals, but these substances found in foods are still very important to good health.
- Poverty and malnutrition go together.

1 What Is Nutrition?

Words to Understand

Excess means extra or too much of something.

A **deficiency** is not enough of something.

Developed countries are those that have advanced industrial, technological, and economic systems.

Developing countries are those that have low industrial, technological, and economic productivity.

Composition refers to what something is made up of.

Legumes are plant foods such as peas and beans that come in pods.

Fiber is the coarse, indigestible material found in plant foods that stimulates the movement of your intestines.

Carbohydrates that are complex have a structure that cannot be broken down as easily by the body's digestive processes.

Something that is **soluble** can be dissolved into water.

To **fortify** a food means to add vitamins or minerals not normally found in it.

Did You Know?

Children and babies need more fat in their diets for their brains and nervous systems to develop. That's why toddlers should drink whole milk, which has more fat, and older kids can drink low-fat or skim milk.

Did You Know?

Food labels will tell you how many grams of fat are in a serving of food. Labels also list the total calories from fat.

Food labels are one way to assess the nutrition levels of the foods you eat.

Nutrition is what we get from the food we eat. It's the part of food that gives our bodies what they need to function—to live and move around, to think and breathe, play and work. Without nutrition, we could not survive for very long.

Malnutrition is when our bodies don't get all the nutrients they need. A person with malnutrition is often more likely to catch diseases. Malnutrition can also affect brain function, eyesight, and the function of various body organs. If a child has malnutrition, she may not grow as tall or weigh as much as would be normal for a child her age. If a pregnant woman is malnourished, the fetus within her may not develop normally.

Nutrients

The food we eat contains different types of nutrients (the materials that supply us with nutrition). These nutrients include calories, carbohydrates, fats, proteins, vitamins, minerals, fiber, and water. We need some of all these; our bodies are healthiest and work their best when they have

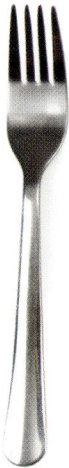

Nutrition Facts
Per 1 meal

Amount	% Daily Value
Calories 0	
Fat 0 g	**0 %**
Carbohydrate 0 g	**0 %**
Protein 0 g	

Not a significant source of saturated fat, trans fat, cholesterol, sodium, fiber, sugars, vitamin A, vitamin C, calcium or iron.

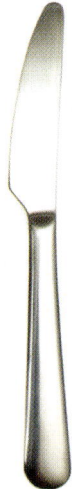

a balanced diet made of different foods that contain all the nutrients.

Most foods contain a mix of some or all of the different kinds of nutrients. Some nutrients are required every day (or nearly every day), while others aren't needed as often. Scientists sometimes sort nutrients into two categories: the macronutrients—the ones we need in large quantities, including carbohydrates, fat, fiber, protein, and water—and the micronutrients—the ones we don't need as much of, such as vitamins and minerals. Poor health can be caused by an imbalance of nutrients, whether an **excess** or a **deficiency**.

The macronutrients (except for fiber and water) provide our bodies with energy. They are the body's fuel, and they contain calories. Vitamins and minerals do not give us energy, but our bodies need them for other reasons.

Calories

If you live in one of the world's **developed** countries, you've probably seen low-calorie foods advertised on television and in magazines as though low-calorie foods were best. It's true that the developed nations of the world have a problem with obesity; in other words, people are eating *too many* calories. But calories themselves aren't bad for you. Your body needs calories for energy. It's only when you eat more calories than you burn off through activity that you begin to gain weight.

Most foods and drinks contain calories. Some foods, such as celery and lettuce, contain very few calories. Other foods, such as peanuts and sugary foods, contain a lot of calories. The nutrition facts labels on food will tell you how many calories are found in the foods you purchase at the store.

The human body comes in many sizes, and each body burns energy at a different rate; this means that everyone needs a different number of calories to be healthy. The recommended calorie range for most teenagers is 1,600 to 3,000 per day. Boys usually need more than girls, and

Did You Know?

Regular weight gain is the most important sign that a child is developing and growing the way he should. Health-care workers usually weigh children regularly. If a child does not gain weight for two months, he may need more food or different types of food than what he is currently getting.

Did You Know?

Breast-feeding is the best way to make sure a baby's nutritional needs are being met during the first six months of life. Children who are breast-fed receive exactly the right amount of nutrients in the right proportions.

people who are very active will need more calories than those who exercise less.

Protein

Most people need about 1 gram (or a third of an ounce) of protein per kilogram of body mass (or about 0.4 grams of protein per pound of body weight)—so if you weigh 50 kilograms (110 pounds), you'll need to eat about 50 grams of protein each day. As a general rule, between 10 percent and 15 percent of your total calories should come from protein, which means if you eat 2,000 calories per day, at least 200 should come from protein. When you eat a balanced diet, it's easy to get the protein you need, but for various reasons, not everyone eats a balanced diet. Junk foods such as chips, cookies, and other snacks are low in protein, so people who get most of their daily calories

Many people in the world's developed nations take for granted that a meal contains protein (meat), carbohydrates (potatoes), and vitamins (green vegetables, tomatoes). In developing nations, however, a meal may be only a carbohydrate such as rice.

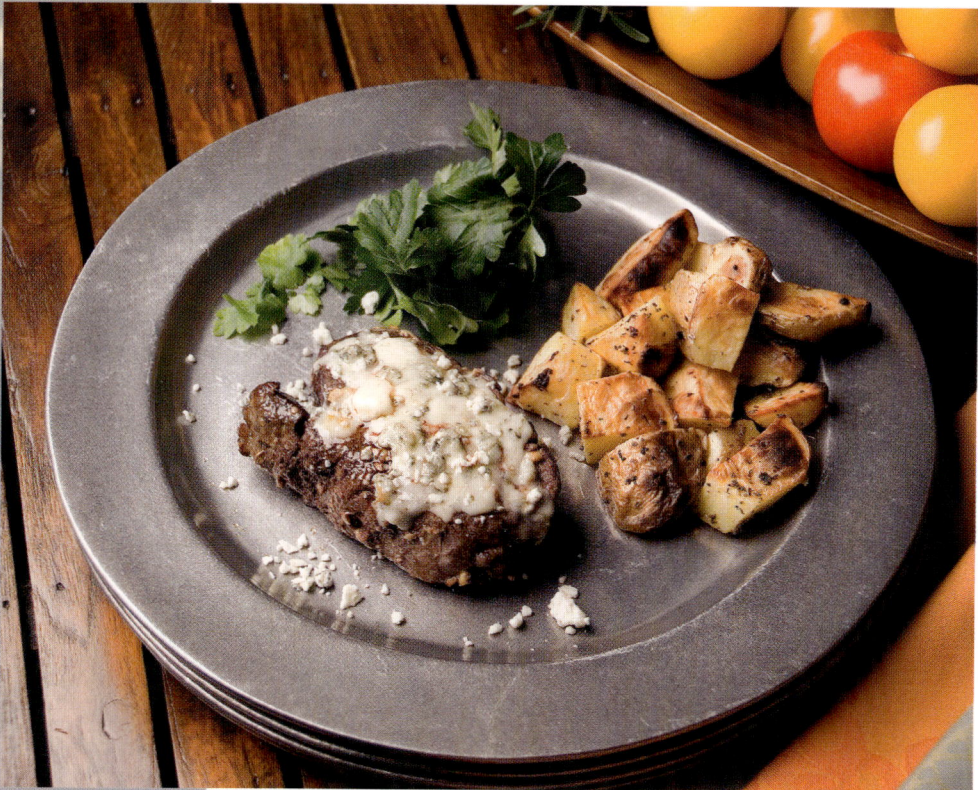

from these sorts of food may not be eating enough protein. Meanwhile, for many people who live in the **developing** world, foods that contain protein are expensive and less plentiful than other foods.

Amino acids are the building blocks of protein. The combination of amino acids is what determines the type of protein. There are two types of protein—animal and plant—but there are about 20 different amino acids, divided between essential amino acids and nonessential ones. Essential means the body cannot make these chemicals on its own and must obtain them from a food source. Good nutrition includes all the amino acids, though, because your body needs them all in order to be healthy.

Depending on the **composition** of amino acids, proteins are either "complete" or "incomplete." Animal protein has all the amino acids your body needs, so beef, chicken, pork, fish, and eggs are all complete proteins. Vegetable proteins—from nuts, seeds, and **legumes**—are usually incomplete, which means they are either missing amino acids or they have too few of them to keep up with what your body needs. Vegetable proteins need to be combined with each other, to make sure all your body's amino acid needs are met.

Carbohydrates

The main fuel your body uses to move around comes from carbohydrates. Carbohydrates can be refined (simple) and unrefined. Refined sugars (such as those found in soft drinks, snack foods, and white bread) have already been broken down by food processing; in other words, machinery has removed all the bits of fiber from the food. Often, refined sugars have been added to the food, instead of being a natural part of it (as is the case with fruit and vegetables). Your body has to work harder to get the energy from unrefined carbohydrates, and these more **complex** carbohydrates are better for you. Good nutrition requires more complex carbohydrates and as few refined carbohydrates as possible.

Did You Know?

If you eat more calories than your body needs, the leftover calories are turned into fat—and too much body fat can lead to health problems.

Did You Know?

Your body needs some calories just to keep your heart beating, your lungs breathing in and out, your digestive system moving food through it, and all the other functions your body does all the time without you even thinking about it.

Did You Know?

Your body burns only about one calorie per minute while watching television, which is about the same as what you burn while you're sleeping.

Whole-grain breads are better for you than white bread. Whole grains have more fiber and complex carbohydrates.

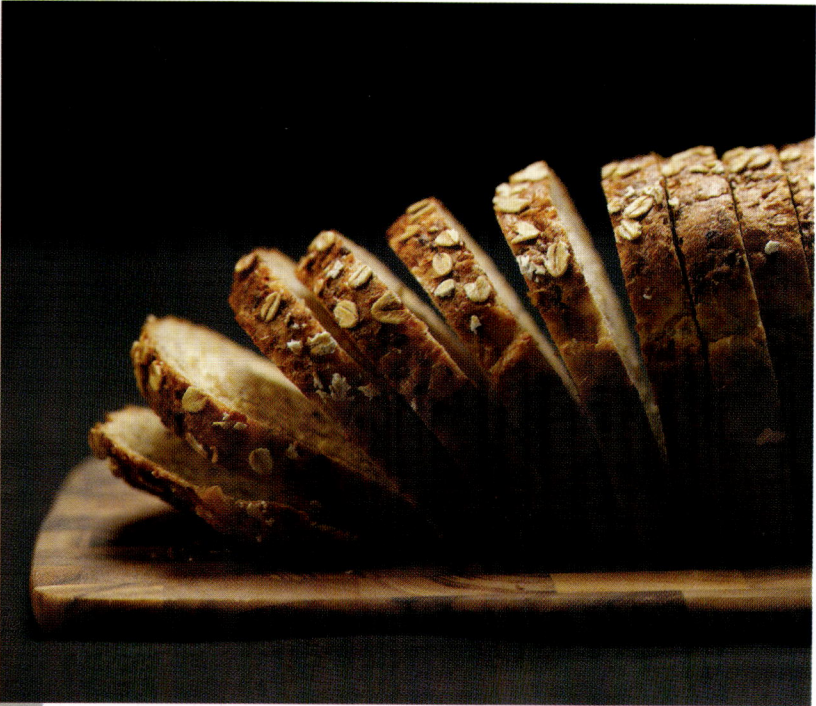

Fats

In many developed countries, fat is talked about as though it were something bad, something we all ought to avoid if at all possible. Although it's true that a high-fat diet is unhealthy and can contribute to a variety of diseases (including heart disease and obesity-related conditions), here's the truth: we need fat in our diets. The right kind of fat in the right amounts is good for you. Fat provides calories that give the body energy; it helps absorb some vitamins; it is one of the building blocks of hormones, special chemicals that give directions to your body; and it insulates your body's nervous system tissue. What's more, the fat in food helps people feel satisfied, so they end up not eating as many calories.

Fat is a normal part of food. Some foods, including most fruits and vegetables, have almost no fat, while other foods, including oils, nuts, and many meats, have plenty of fat. You need to eat fat every day to be healthy. Teenagers and adults need to get about 30 percent of their daily calories from fat. This means that if you eat about 2,000 calories every day, 600 of those calories should come from fat.

Unsaturated fat is the kind of fat that is best for you. It is found in plant foods and fish. Olive oil, peanut oil, canola oil, albacore tuna, and salmon are all good sources of unsaturated fat.

Saturated fats are found in meat and other animal products, such as dairy products (except those made from skim milk). Saturated fats are also in palm and coconut oils, which are often used in the baked goods you buy at the store. Eating too much saturated fat can increase your risk of heart disease.

Trans fats are found in margarine, especially the sticks, and in many of the snack foods, baked goods, and fried foods you buy at stores and restaurants. Trans fats are also listed on the food label. Like saturated fats, trans fats can raise cholesterol and increase the risk of heart disease.

Vitamins

Your body doesn't need as large quantities of vitamins as it does proteins, carbohydrates, and fats, but if you don't get enough of the right vitamins, your nutrition will suffer—and you will not function as well either mentally and physically. Your body does not make vitamins, so you have

Did You Know?

A calorie is a unit used to measure food's energy. When we're talking about nutrition, the word "calorie" is usually used instead of the more precise scientific term "kilocalorie," which is the amount of energy required to raise the temperature of a liter of water one degree centigrade at sea level. Most people say "calorie" when they're talking about food energy, but it is actually a kilocalorie: 1000 true calories of energy.

Sample Meal with the Right Percentage of Fat

Two slices of bread = 13% fat (30 of 230 calories from fat)
Two tablespoons of peanut butter = 75% fat (140 of 190 calories from fat)
One tablespoon of jelly = 0% fat (0 of 50 calories from fat)
One cup of 1% milk = 18 % (20 of 110 calories from fat)
Apple = 0% (0 of 80 calories from fat)
Total = 29% fat (190 of 660 calories from fat)

Did You Know?

Each gram of carbohydrate or protein provides the body with 4 calories, while each gram of fat provides 9 calories.

Did You Know?

An easy way to figure out how much protein you need is to take your weight in pounds, divide it in half, and subtract 10. The total will be the number of grams of protein you should eat each day. For concentrated proteins such as meat, a 4-ounce serving (about 125 grams) is about the size of a computer mouse or your fist.

to get them from food. Not having enough of one vitamin can affect your body's ability to absorb other vitamins. Each vitamin has a role to play to keep us healthy.

Vitamins that are fat-**soluble** can be stored in your body for a while—some for days, others for months. This means your body can build up a supply to keep on hand for when they are needed. Vitamins A, D, E, and K are fat-soluble. Meanwhile, water-soluble vitamins—vitamins C and B—travel through your bloodstream to your kidneys, where they pass into your urine, and eventually leave your body when you go to the toilet. Your body uses what it needs while the vitamins are traveling through your system. Since you don't have the ability to store them for later, these vitamins need to be replaced often (by eating foods that contain them).

Here are some of the most important vitamins your body needs for good nutrition:

- *The B vitamins* (found in beans, peas, and whole-grain foods) help your body make energy. They support the creation of red blood cells, which carry oxygen around your body.

- *Vitamin C* (found in oranges and other citrus fruit, tomatoes, cabbage, and red and green peppers) helps your body's tissues (for example, skin and muscles) keep healthy. It also helps cuts and wounds to heal and helps you ward off illnesses.

- *Vitamin D* (found in milk, eggs, and salmon) helps you build strong bones and teeth by helping you take in the calcium you need. Regular sunlight helps your body take in vitamin D, but people who live in certain areas of the world may not be exposed to sunshine for long periods of the year. Many developed nations **fortify** milk with vitamin D.

- *Vitamin E* (found in nuts, spinach, and sardines) helps keep body tissues such as your eyes and skin healthy. It also protects your lungs from being damaged by polluted air, and it helps in the making of red blood cells.

• *Vitamin K* (found in liver, pork, and yogurt) helps your blood clot when you bleed, so that the blood flow does not continue. Some foods with vitamin K include pork, liver, and yogurt.

• *Vitamin A* (found in carrots, pumpkin, yellow squash, apricots, and eggs) is good for your eyes. It helps you to see better at night, and it also helps you see colors. A severe lack of vitamin A can even cause blindness. Few people have such an extreme lack of vitamin A; they may not even notice that they aren't getting enough of this vitamin, but their ability to fight off diseases will be decreased.

If you eat a variety of vegetables each day, you can be sure you're getting all the vitamins your body needs.

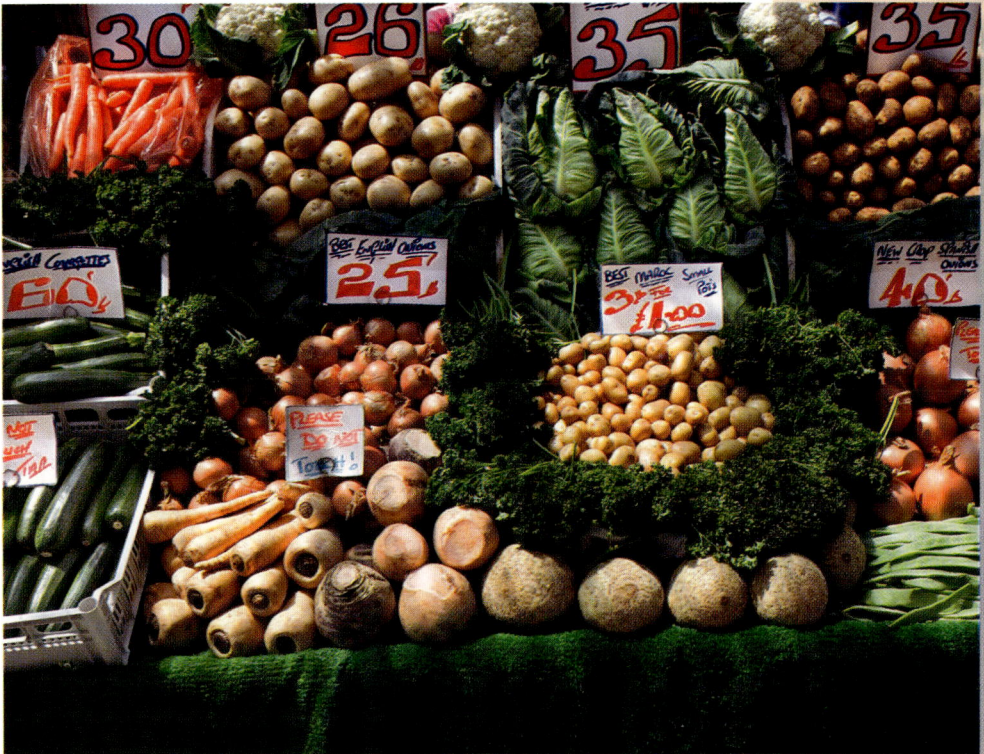

24789 Dewdney Trunk Road
Maple Ridge, B.C.
V4R 1X2

Did You
Know?

*Eggs are the
most ideal
protein. They're
the standard to
which all other
protein foods
are measured
in terms of
"usability" by the
body.*

Minerals

Minerals are the chemicals found in metals and in the soil. It may seem strange that your body needs something like iron (the same substance that's use to manufacture steel for cars and machinery) or copper (found in coins and cooking pots)—but it does! Your body needs only very tiny bits of minerals like these, but those tiny bits are important for good nutrition. You don't eat coins or metal pots, of course (and too much of many minerals could be dangerous to your health), so how do you get minerals inside your body?

First, plants take in minerals from the soil—and you get those minerals from eating plants. Animals also eat the plants, and the minerals enter their bodies, so you can also get some minerals from eating meat. Minerals can be present in water as well. How much and what minerals you take into your body will depend on how much of a mineral is present in the soil in the region where your food, water, or meat comes from. Many developed nations add minerals to their foods, so not getting enough of these substances is seldom a concern, as long as you're eating a balanced diet. If you live in a developing nation, you may be dependent on the food that grows on the land where

Water

Anything that's alive—from tiny one-celled creatures to human beings to trees—needs water in order to live. Water makes up more than half of a human's body weight and a person can't survive for more than a few days without it. When your body doesn't have enough water, that's called being dehydrated. Low-level dehydration can affect your body and mind's performance, while a bad case of dehydration can make you sick. When your urine is very dark yellow, it's means your body is holding on to water, so it's probably time to drink more. You need extra water when you exercise and when it's hot out. People who live in developed nations may take water for granted (turn on the faucet and out it comes), but people who live in other regions of the world may have to walk long distances and carry water back to their home.

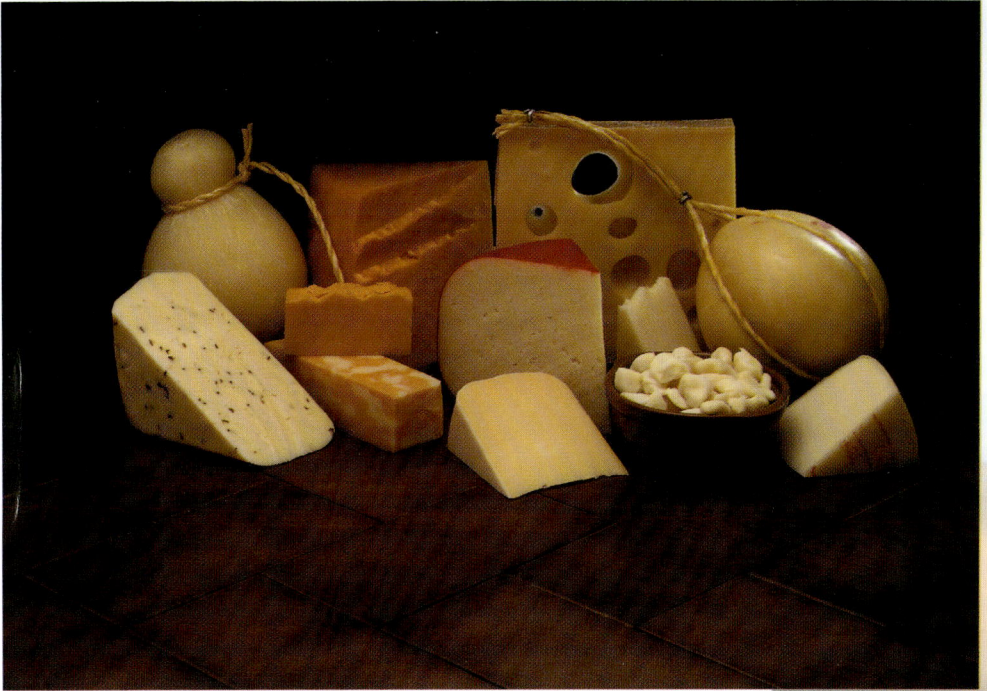

you live, which may or may not have all the minerals you need for good nutrition.

Here are some of the minerals most important to good nutrition:

- *Calcium* (found in dairy products, tofu, and cabbage) is needed to help build your bones and teeth.

- *Sodium* (the mineral found in salt) helps regulate the fluid balance in your body; it also helps your muscles expand (stretch) and contract (get smaller), which is what allows your body to move. Salt is present in all your body's fluids, including tears and sweat. You may have heard that a low-salt diet is often considered to be healthy, and too much salt can cause high-blood pressure—but not enough salt can also be dangerous to your health.

All kinds of cheese are good sources of protein and calcium. Many of them also have high levels of saturated fat, though, so you need to be careful of how much you eat.

Did You Know?

You don't have to eat all your amino acids every day. Good nutrition for children and young adults means they need to eat a complete assortment of amino acids every week. Adults don't need to get all the amino acids as often, but over the course of a month, they should be sure to eat the full range of amino acids.

Did You Know?

Watch the fat content in the protein foods you eat. Choose lean meats and non-fat dairy products to limit your fat intake—but don't eliminate carbohydrates and fat altogether, as this imbalance can damage your health.

• *Iron* (found in dark, leafy vegetables and peanuts) helps your brain develop normally.

• *Iodine* is also important for normal brain development. A lack of iodine can cause goiters (where a part of the body called the thyroid gland becomes larger), hearing and speaking difficulty, and poor growth. The world's developed nations add iodine to their salt to make sure that people get enough of this mineral, and nearly two-thirds of the developing nations also add iodine to salt.

Food and Finances

Everyone on Earth needs good nutrition, but not all people get the foods they need to be healthy. Sometimes poor nutrition is caused by bad eating habits—getting too many calories from high-fat, sugary foods that contribute to obesity and don't contain enough of the nutrients our bodies need. In many parts of the world, though, both in developed and developing nations, poor nutrition is linked to poverty. Families that don't have enough money may not be able to afford a healthy variety of foods. In some parts of the world, there simply may not be enough food resources to meet the needs of the communities who live there. Poverty looks different in different parts of the world—but it always has an enormous impact on nutrition.

The Food Pyramid

The United States' Food Guide Pyramid is a picture people use to help them understand how to eat healthy. The colored stripes represent the main food groups.

orange = grains
green = vegetables
red = fruits
yellow = fats and oils

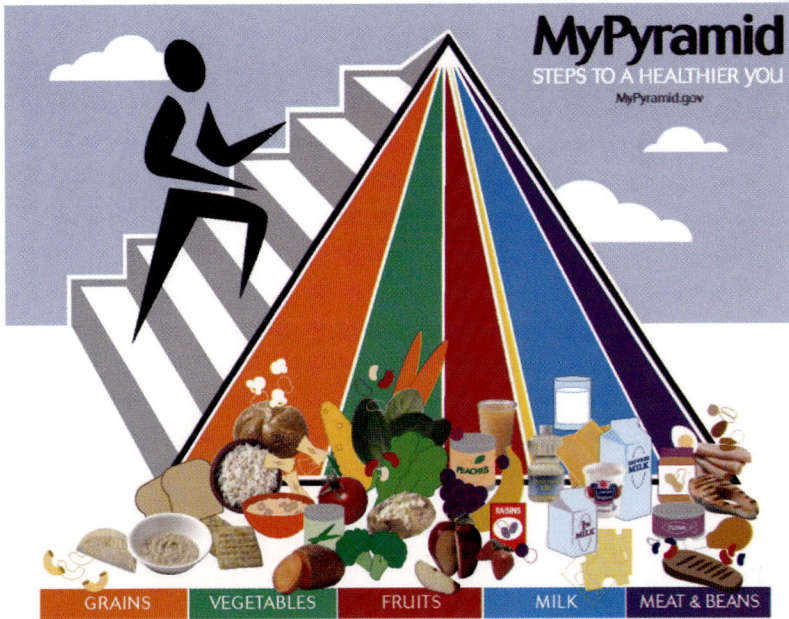

The U.S. Food Pyramid.

blue = milk and dairy products
purple = meat, beans, fish, and nuts

Here are the important things you should learn from the pyramid:

- **Eat a variety of foods.** A balanced diet is one that includes all the food groups, so eat foods from every color, every day.

- **Eat less of some foods, and more of others.** Notice that the stripes for meat and protein (purple) and oils (yellow) are skinnier than the others. That's because you need less of those foods than you do of fruits, vegetables, grains, and dairy foods. You can also see that the stripes start out wider at the bottom of the pyramid and get thinner as they reach the top. That's meant to show you that not all foods are created equal, even within a healthy food group like fruit. For instance, an apple tart would probably be in that thin part of the fruit stripe because it has

Did You Know?

Athletes and other people who exercise a lot have different nutritional needs than those who don't. They need both more protein and more carbohydrates.

Nutrition and Health Around the World

• About 30% of children in many developed countries, including Canada, Australia, New Zealand, and the United States, are either overweight or obese as result of poor nutrition habits.

• Over 70% of preschool children in India are estimated to be iron-deficient. (In other words, they don't get enough iron to be healthy.)

• In Canada, fewer than 5% of pregnant women know that vitamin supplements would contribute to the health of their unborn children.

• About 70% of children under 6 in Kenya suffer from vitamin A deficiency.

• As many as 18 million low-birth-weight babies are born every year due to malnutrition; that's 14% of all live births. These children are likely to suffer from infections, weakened immunity, learning disabilities, and impaired physical and mental development.

(Source: UNICEF International Web site)

Did You Know?

Most Americans get about 50 percent of their carbohydrates from simple, refined sugars. Over the course of a year, the average American drinks 54 gallons of soda, which contains the highest amounts of added sugars of any food.

added sugar and fat. A whole apple would be down in the wide part because you can eat more of those within a healthy diet.

Global Images for Good Nutrition

The United States represents a balanced, healthy diet with a pyramid, but many governments around the world choose different shapes to teach people the right way to eat. The World Health Organization (WHO), along with the UN's Food and Agriculture Organization (FAO), hold conferences on health concerns such as malnutrition and obesity. Governments around the world look to these international organizations for the latest, and most accurate, nutritional guidelines. These guidelines are adapted by various governments for their various cultural diets and traditional eating habits. The UN's FAO and the WHO lead the way for countries around the world to give the very best nutritional information to their people, so that

Japan's Spinning Food Top.

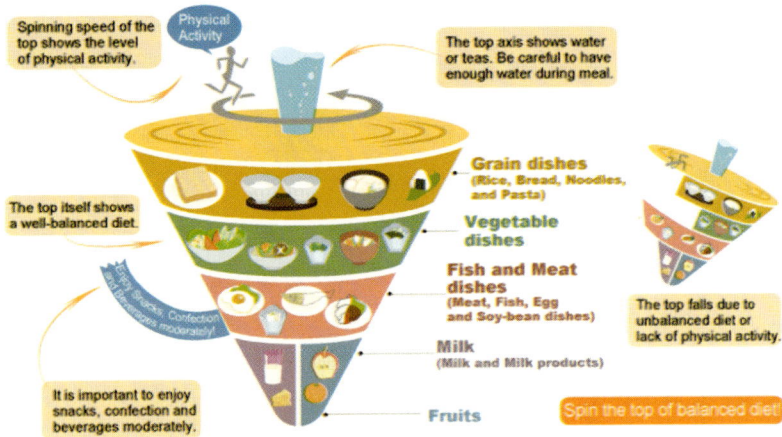

Spinning speed of the top shows the level of physical activity.

Physical Activity

The top axis shows water or teas. Be careful to have enough water during meal.

The top itself shows a well-balanced diet.

Grain dishes (Rice, Bread, Noodles, and Pasta)

Vegetable dishes

Fish and Meat dishes (Meat, Fish, Egg and Soy-bean dishes)

The top falls due to unbalanced diet or lack of physical activity.

Milk (Milk and Milk products)

Enjoy snacks, Confection and beverages moderately!

It is important to enjoy snacks, confection and beverages moderately.

Fruits

Spin the top of balanced diet!

they may make the best food choices they can. The WHO is committed to maintaining health worldwide, and good nutrition is a key part of that. Countries around the world use many different methods to get this information to their citizens.

A rainbow symbolizes Canadian guidelines. Among its recommendations are to eat five to twelve servings of grains and up to ten daily servings of fruits and vegetables. They also advise moderation in the use of caffeine. A pyramid represents Chile's nutritional recommendations. When the government first began issuing guidelines more than ten years ago, the emphasis was on solving its malnutrition problem. Today's goal is to help combat the country's growing problem of obesity. Recommenda-

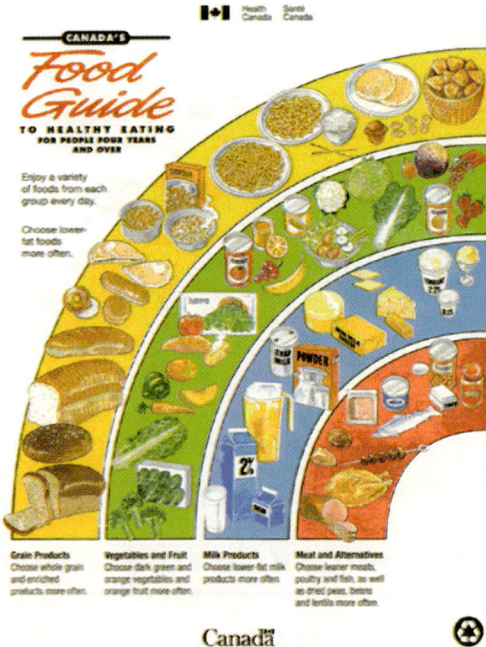

Health Canada's Food Rainbow.

Health Canada   Santé Canada

CANADA'S

Food Guide

TO HEALTHY EATING
FOR PEOPLE FOUR YEARS AND OVER

Enjoy a variety of foods from each group every day.

Choose lower-fat foods more often.

Grain Products
Choose whole grain and enriched products more often.

Vegetables and Fruit
Choose dark green and orange vegetables and orange fruit more often.

Milk Products
Choose lower-fat milk products more often.

Meat and Alternatives
Choose leaner meats, poultry and fish, as well as dried peas, beans and lentils more often.

Canada

Real People
Iron Deficiency in Laos

Vanhdy and Soudsadi Keothaune have had four children together, but fourteen years ago Soudsadi suffered from iodine deficiency. The delivery of her firstborn was difficult and her child's physical and mental development was slow.

Nine years ago a survey of school children in Laos found that 95% suffered from iodine deficiency. But there has been progress battling the problem through salt iodization. In 1993, Laos was listed as one of the countries whose population was most affected by iodine deficiency. Now, things are different. Laos is now projected to be the first country in the region after China to achieve universal salt iodization.

Vanhdy and Soudsadi have seen the improvements in their children. "Our second child is taller than the first child. Videth has more creativity, and also more ideas." There are still 20% of hard-to-reach households without iodized salt, and people have to guard against imported salt from other countries where manufacturers falsely claim the salt is iodized.

(Source: UNICEF International Web site)

tions include consuming low-fat milk products and lean meats. Meanwhile, France recommends enjoying three good meals every day. It also suggests monthly weigh-ins to keep tabs on the results of those good meals! Costa Rica's nutritional guidelines are presented on a plate, and they advise that foods be consumed in the most natural

Vegetarians must eat "complementary" vegetable proteins to make a single complete protein source. For example, they need to eat beans with rice—or a rice cake with peanut butter or hummus (made from seeds). Soy is a good, low-fat source of protein for vegetarians. Most protein bars and protein powders use soy protein, casein, or whey as their base, which are all are complete proteins. Whey, however, is a milk product, so if you are a vegan, you may want to avoid products that contain whey.

form possible. Australia and Great Britain also use plates as their food guide visual aide. In Indonesia, people are encouraged to eat breakfast every day, and individuals are advised to eat iron-rich foods, consume about one-half of their daily calories from complex carbohydrates such as whole grains, and use iodized salt rather than sea salt. A spinning top is the nutritional symbol of Japan's guidelines. According to Japanese guidelines, happy eating means a happy family life, and they encourage family meal preparation and eating. They also suggest using vegetable oil rather than animal fats. Variety is also important in the Japanese diet, and the guidelines recommend consuming thirty different foods every day.

Although culture plays a role in how a country talks about good nutrition, all nations agree that nutrition builds strong countries, one individual at a time. No matter how many government programs encourage good nutrition, however, and how many times you learn about it in school, ultimately, good nutrition is up to you.

Did You Know?

Getting enough iron is especially important for children between the ages of six months and two years. In developed countries, many infant foods such as cereals have added iron, and 49 of the world's countries fortify their flour with iron.

STRAIGHT FROM THE SOURCE

(by Kent Page, UNICEF)

Community Gardens Provide Food, Income for Families

AGADEZ, Niger, 14 September 2005—Niger is struggling to cope with a nutrition crisis. But in the village of Alikinkin, community gardens are an oasis of beauty and a source of food, helping children avoid the worst effects of the crisis.

In Alikinkin's gardens, donkeys, goats and birds flourish among the grasses, bushes, palm and date trees. Neatly planted rows of crops are irrigated with fresh water pumped from wells—a stark contrast to the situation in other parts of the country.

UNICEF's office in Agadez, a town near Alikinkin, is supporting 50 community garden projects by helping construct water wells, providing gardening seeds, fertilizer, insecticide, fencing and tools.

The goal is to ensure that village children have access to nutritious foods. The gardens produce tomatoes, onions, carrots, peas, beans, cabbage, potatoes and wheat.

What Do You Think?

- How are gardens and nutrition connected?

- Do you think your nutrition concerns are similar to those of the people who live in Alikinkin in Niger? Why or why not?

- Do you think it would be better if developed nations merely shipped their excess food to Niger (instead of helping to build gardens) to ensure good nutrition for communities like Alikinkin? Why or why not?

Find Out More

Food Guidelines by Country
http://www.fao.org/ag/agn/nutrition/education_
guidelines_country_en.stm

MyPyramid
www.mypyramid.gov

U.S. Department of Agriculture, Center for Nutrition Policy and Promotion
www.cnpp.usda.gov

Here's what you need to know

- Good nutrition is necessary at every developmental stage.
- During adolescence, the growth rate is extremely fast, requiring increased levels of some nutrients.

Words to Understand

Developmental stage refers to a distinct phase in an individual's maturation.

Immunity is your body's ability to fight off certain diseases or other harmful invaders.

Osteoporosis is when a person's bones become brittle and break easily because they lose some essential components.

Puberty is the stage of becoming physically capable of sexual reproduction.

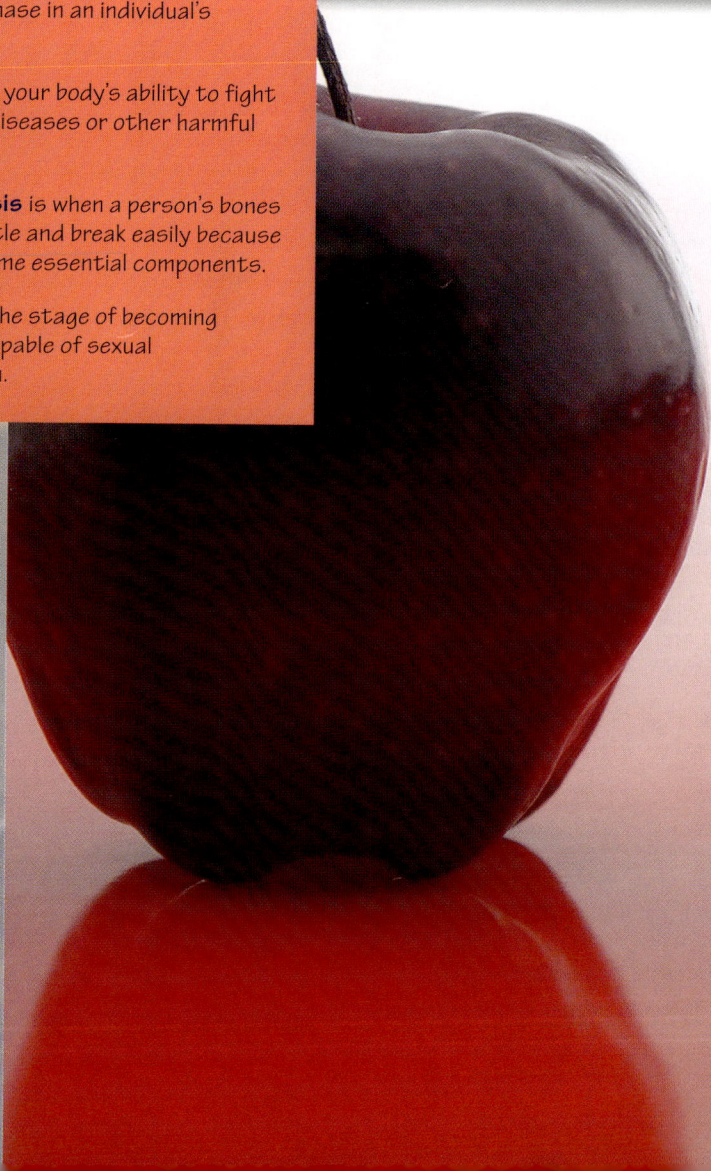

2

Nutrition and Young People

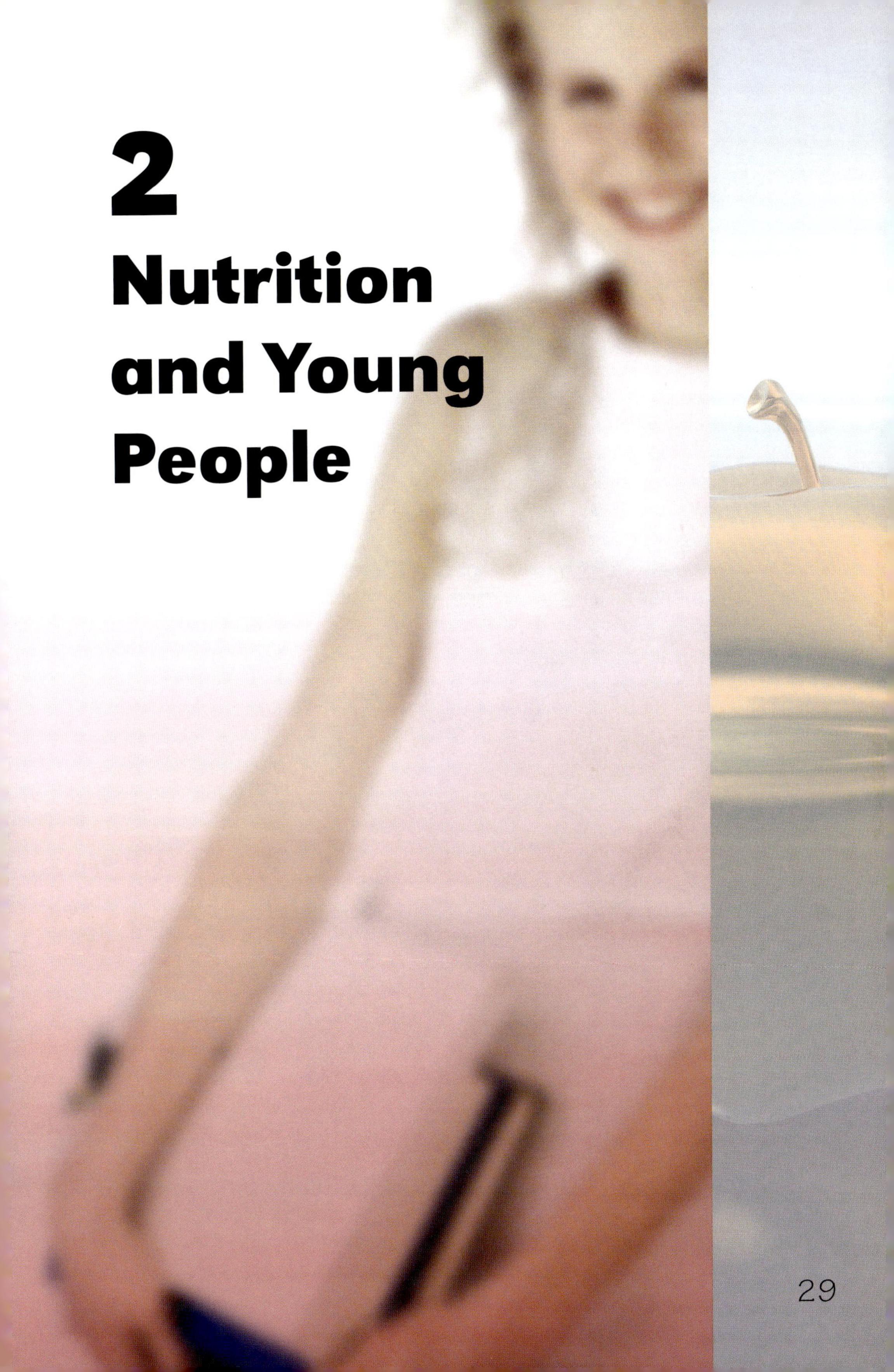

A tree may be one of nature's sturdiest creations. But a tree wasn't always big and strong; it was once a seed and a sapling before becoming strong and tall enough to support a swing or a tree house. As it matured, it needed nutrients that would eventually allow it to become a healthy, full-grown tree.

Early Nutrition

As with the tree, the human body needs proper nutrients to grow into a healthy, strong adult. At each **developmental stage**, nutrition is the building block that leads to a healthy adult body. Most experts believe that the first two years of life are most important in setting the stage for healthy growth. Inadequate nutrition during that time may lead to problems in mental and motor development.

Good nutrition is especially important for young children whose bodies are growing and developing so quickly. What's more, the habits of a lifetime are often begun very early in childhood.

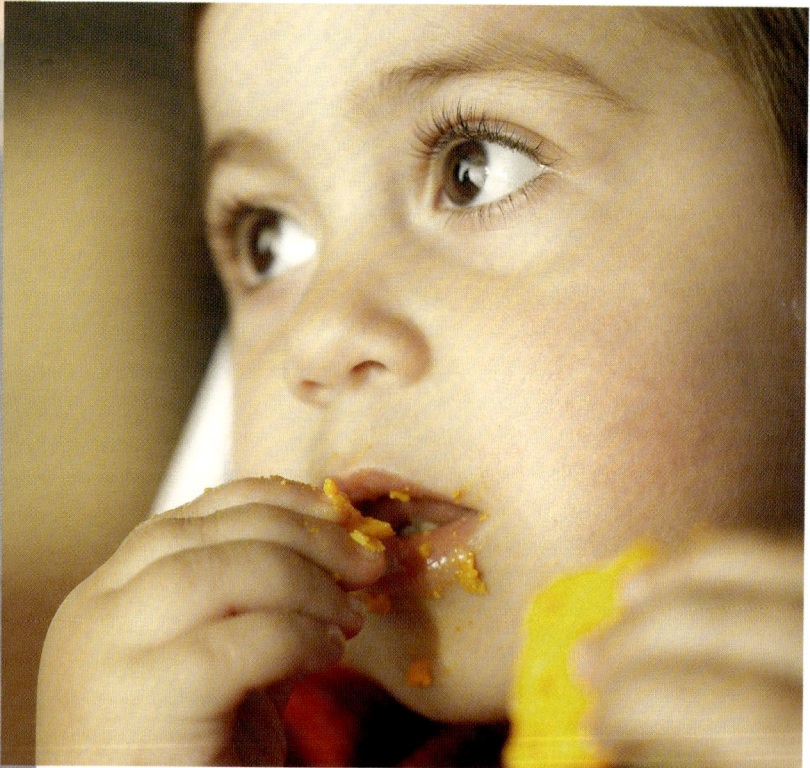

The WHO encourages breast-feeding for the first six months of life. Not only does the baby receive nourishment from its mother's milk, the mother's antibodies pass through the milk, providing the baby with **immunity** against some diseases. A growing body of scientific research also indicates breast-fed babies may not be as likely to develop childhood obesity as those who are not breast fed. Mothers are encouraged to continue breast-feeding until the child is two years old, adding solids and additional liquids as needed, especially those that are iron fortified. Fats are crucial in children under age two. They are important in the formation of nerve and brain tissue, so reduced-fat milk and milk products are not recommended for this age group.

Once the child is over age two, dietary needs are not unlike those of adults. Making certain that the child receives adequate nutrition is not always easy, however. Children may be reluctant to try new foods. Others may be happy eating only one or two things; they don't care that every country's dietary guidelines recommend eating a variety of foods! Despite their pickiness when it come to food, most children between ages six and twelve grow one to two feet and double their weight. If they don't, it could be a sign of undernutrition, which requires medical intervention. But in most cases, these are passing phases, and no harm comes from them, though doctors may recommend a multivitamin as a precaution.

Nutrition During Adolescence

During adolescence, most teens experience an increased growth rate. Increased nutritional needs are required to support this growth period. If increased nutritional needs are not met, delays in maturation may occur. According to research, nutritional habits developed during this time may help prevent nutrition-related diseases in the future. For example, an adolescent who consumes a diet low in red meat and high in vegetables, especially certain greens, may help stave off some forms of heart disease and cancer.

Before **puberty**, there is little difference in the dietary needs of males and females. But puberty brings body changes, and with them, the nutritional needs of boys and girls begin to differentiate. For example, girls begin to menstruate and need additional iron in their diets. Besides gender, nutritional needs are based on factors such as activity level and rate of growth. In general, males require more calories than females because they have a higher growth rate. This is also reflected in the recommended caloric intake for males and females. The Food and Nutrition Board of the United States recommends total caloric intake of 2,200/day for females between the ages of eleven and twenty-four. For males between eleven and fourteen, it recommends 2,500/day; for males age fifteen to eighteen, it recommends 3,000/day, but reduces caloric intake to 2,900 for males between nineteen and twenty-four. Adolescents and their families need to be aware of their changing nutritional requirements.

Many teenagers are fond of fast food, including burgers and fries. Although it's okay to eat this kind of food once in a while, keep in mind that these foods are high in fat. Although they also contain protein and carbohydrates, they are usually very low in vitamins.

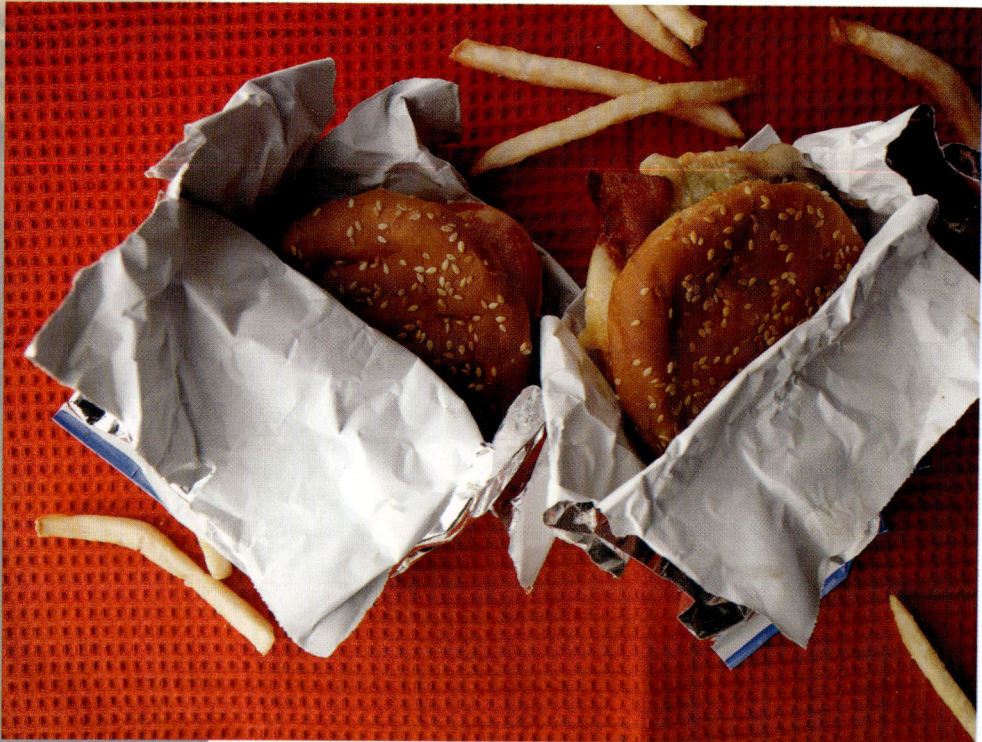

Protein

The amount of protein required increases during teens' peak growing periods. In general, females' peak growth occurs between ages eleven and fourteen; for boys, peak growth is between fifteen and eighteen. Protein can be found in meat, fish, eggs, and other meat and dairy products. Also, many beans and nuts contain the proteins essential to health. The WHO/FAO recommendations for protein intake change with age, increasing as people get older. For example, a baby of two months needs 1.82 grams per kilogram of body weight per day. At six years old, however, that requirement is 19.7 g/kg of body weight per day. Protein is essential for the body's growth and structures. These structures include fingernails, hair, cell membranes, and enzymes, which break down food.

Carbohydrates

Though carbohydrates are found in fruit, vegetables, and whole grains, some teens get many of their carbs from sugar and sugary foods and drinks. Though it might provide an energy boost, the benefits are short-lived, and the calories added may lead to undesirable weight gain. For long-term energy, complex carbohydrates, such as those found in vegetables and whole grains, are more efficient.

Fat

Some fat is necessary for good health, but the type of fat consumed does make a difference. The Dietary Guidelines for Americans suggests that no more than 30 percent of an adolescent's daily caloric intake be from fats, with no more than 10 percent of that coming from saturated fat.

Some animal fat is actually beneficial, however. Omega-3 fatty acid, found in fish such as salmon and some plants, has proven to be heart and brain healthy. Research has

Ask the Doctor

Q: I've heard that palm oil and other tropical oils raise cholesterol. So why doesn't the label list the cholesterol content per serving?

The reason is that there is no cholesterol in these oils. Cholesterol is found only in animal products. Palm oil will not result in a higher cholesterol level.

Did You Know?

Men can develop osteoporosis, though it is not as well known as it is in women. They need to maintain adequate calcium levels as well.

shown that individuals can benefit from at least one fish meal a week.

Minerals and Vitamins

During adolescence, it is important to increase consumption of calcium. Most adolescents experience 45 percent of bone mass development during this time. Research has shown that adequate calcium intake during this period can help prevent the development of osteoporosis. The recommended daily intake of calcium is 1,300mg/day for those between nine and eighteen. Milk and other dairy products, as well as some vegetables, are the primary sources of calcium.

Another important mineral for teens experiencing a growth peak is iron. When females begin to menstruate, they need additional iron. Between the ages of nine and thirteen, the recommended intake of iron is 8mg/day. For males between the ages of fourteen and eighteen, their peak growth period, it is 11mg/day. Between fourteen and eighteen, it is recommended that girls consume 15mg/day of iron. Iron is readily available in meat, fish, and poultry, as well as in some grains.

In adolescence, zinc plays a role in sexual maturation. Zinc is found in red meat, shellfish, and whole grains.

Vitamins are also important in adolescence. Vitamin A is important in vision, reproduction, and immune function. Blindness can occur with a vitamin A deficiency. According to a study by the U.S. National Academy of Sciences, up to 500,000 children living in developing countries become blind because of a lack of vitamin A. Vitamin A can be found in cereal, milk, carrots, and margarine.

Vitamin C helps in the development of connective tissue. The recommended intake of vitamin C is 45mg/day for those between nine and thirteen, and 75mg/day for males and 65mg/day for females between the ages of fourteen and eighteen. Vitamin C is commonly found in citrus fruit and vegetables.

Folate is found in cereal, orange juice, and bread. It

Real People

Besides being a period of physical growth, adolescence is also a time of exploration. For some, that includes exploring dietary options. Some teens, such as Melissa Hicks, choose vegetarianism. Melissa became a vegetarian when she was fifteen years old. A friend was a vegetarian, and she wanted to try it. At first, she included eggs and dairy products in her diet, but over the years, she has eliminated most of these products. Melissa's mother was supportive, although doubtful since Melissa liked so few vegetables, but her father was concerned about her health. A call to the doctor assured him it was a healthy decision. The family even took a vegetarian cooking class together.

When Melissa first became vegetarian, she did miss some foods—a lot. But she still was still able to eat out with friends. When they got together for pizza, they ordered half cheese and half whatever the others wanted. Now that she's more vegan, Melissa generally orders her own pizza without cheese.

Melissa laughs that people always worry "about what to feed the vegetarian at Thanksgiving." Melissa says she is happy to fill up on side dishes, though she has to ask how they're prepared. Things that might seem to be vegetarian might not be.

plays a major role in DNA and RNA. The recommended intake is up to 400 micrograms (µg) per day.

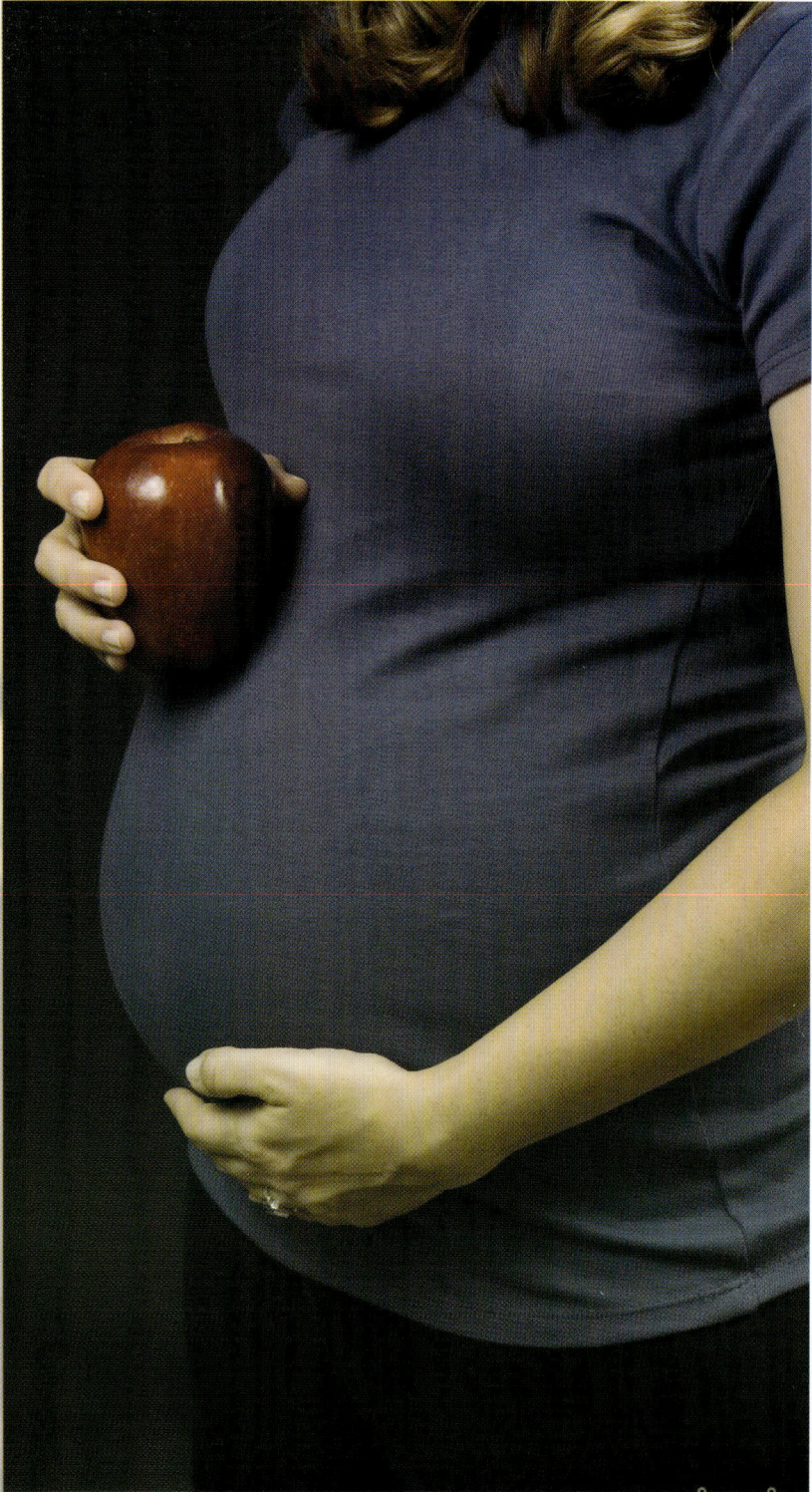

Diet plays an important role in the healthy development of an unborn child. Researchers have found that folic acid is particularly important as a supplement to all pregnant women's diets, as it prevents birth defects.

Nutritional Needs in the Later Years

As one ages, nutritional needs change. For example, during people's twenties and thirties, they are encouraged to increase intake of iron and calcium. If they are considering pregnancy, women are encouraged to consume folic acid. During their forties, individuals become more prone to high cholesterol, type 2 diabetes, high blood pressure, and other nutrition-related conditions. High-fiber and lower-fat foods are recommended, as are foods high in potassium, such as bananas. B vitamins and calcium are especially important in the fifties and beyond. Antioxidants play an important role in preventing heart disease as well as some vision problems.

Ultimately, good nutrition is vital to everyone. It plays an important role in fighting off disease.

Garibaldi Secondary School
24789 Dewdney Trunk Road
Maple Ridge, B.C.
V4R 1X2

STRAIGHT FROM THE SOURCE

(From the WHO document Public Health Nutrition, "Nutrition-Friendly Schools Initiative.")

Nutrition and Schools

Nutrition-related health problems in children are increasingly significant causes of disability and premature death worldwide. While undernutrition continues to be a major problem in many developing countries, the problems of overweight and obesity have reached epidemic proportions globally, and both developed and developing countries are seriously affected. In some countries, the epidemic of obesity sits alongside continuing problems of undernutrition, creating a double burden of nutrition-related ill health among the population, including children. Based on the principle that effectively addressing the increasing global public health problem of the double burden of nutrition-related ill health requires common policy options, the Nutrition-Friendly Schools Initiative (NFSI) has been developed as follow-up to the WHO Expert Meeting on Childhood Obesity (Kobe, 20–24 June 2005).

The main aim of the NFSI is to provide a framework for designing integrated school-based intervention programmes which address the double burden of nutrition related ill health, building on and interconnecting the ongoing work of various agencies and partners. These include the FRESH Initiative, Essential Package (UNICEF/WFP), Child-Friendly Schools (UNICEF), Health-Promoting Schools (WHO), and School Food and Nutrition Education programmes (FAO), to mention just a few. NFSI applies the concept and principles of the Baby-friendly Hospital Initiative (BFHI). Improving the nutritional status of school-aged children is an effective investment for the future generation. Preschools and schools offer many opportunities to promote healthy dietary and physical activity patterns for children, and are also a potential access point for engaging parents and community members in preventing child malnutrition in all its forms (i.e., undernutrition, micronutrient deficiencies, and obesity and other nutrition-related chronic diseases). The universality of the school setting for gaining access to children makes it highly relevant to global efforts to combat the increasing public health problems of the double burden of nutrition-related ill health.

What Do You Think?

- What is meant by the phrase "the double burden of nutrition-related ill health?"

- Do you think schools should be an important part of encouraging healthy eating in children and young adults?

- What is the difference between malnutrition and undernutrition?

Find Out More

To find out more about nutrition and young adults, check out these Web sites:

Eat Your Vegetables
www.k-state.edu/media/webzine/0102/veggies.html

Fruits and Veggies Matter
www.fruitsandveggiesmatter.gov

WHO Department for Nutrition and Development
www.who.int/nutrition/e

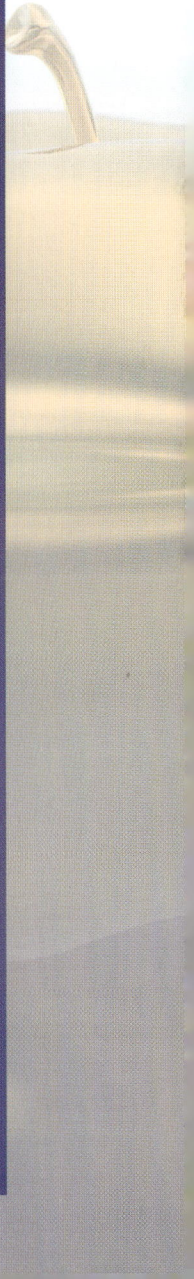

Here's what you need to know

- Nutrition plays a vital role in fighting off disease.
- An athlete's dietary needs vary in some ways from those of a nonathlete.

Words to Understand

Anemia is a condition in which there is a reduced number of red blood cells (the part of your blood that carries oxygen to your other body cells).

The **immune system** consists of the organs, glands, and tissues that work together to help protect the body from harmful foreign substances.

Antiretroviral medications are used to treat infections caused by retroviruses, especially HIV.

Electrolytes are chemical compounds that separate into ions in a solution and are able to conduct electricity.

3

Nutrition and Your Body

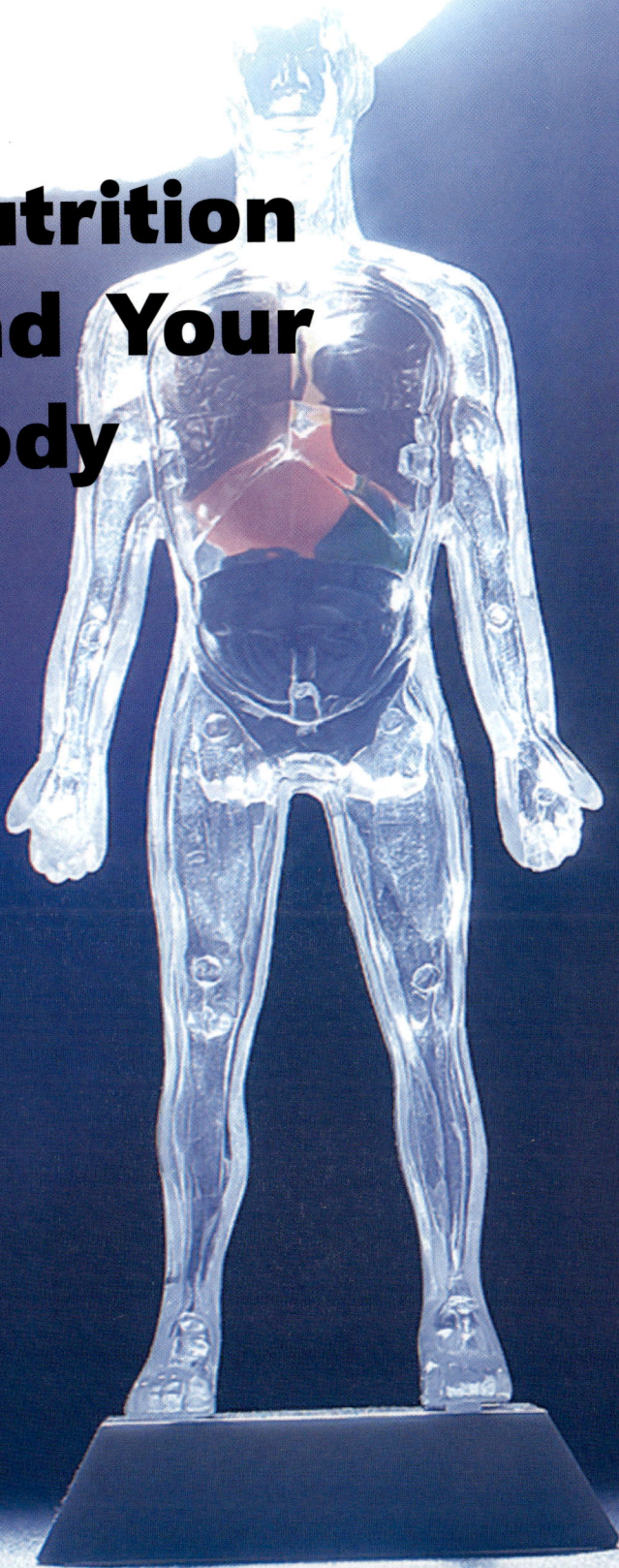

Nutrition doesn't only provide fuel for the body to grow and run efficiently; it also helps fight off disease and illness. In addition, good nutrition can also help treat some physical conditions. In chapter 2, we learned that doses of vitamin A can prevent a form of blindness. Iron supplements are used to treat anemia. But research has opened doors to other ways nutrition may play a role in health.

Nutrition and the Immune System

The body's basic weapon against disease and illness is the immune system. A body that is undernourished will not have the tools it needs to build the blood cells to fight off disease. According to UNICEF, "More than half of all child deaths are associated with malnutrition, which

Poor nutrition may make these African children more susceptible to a variety of diseases.

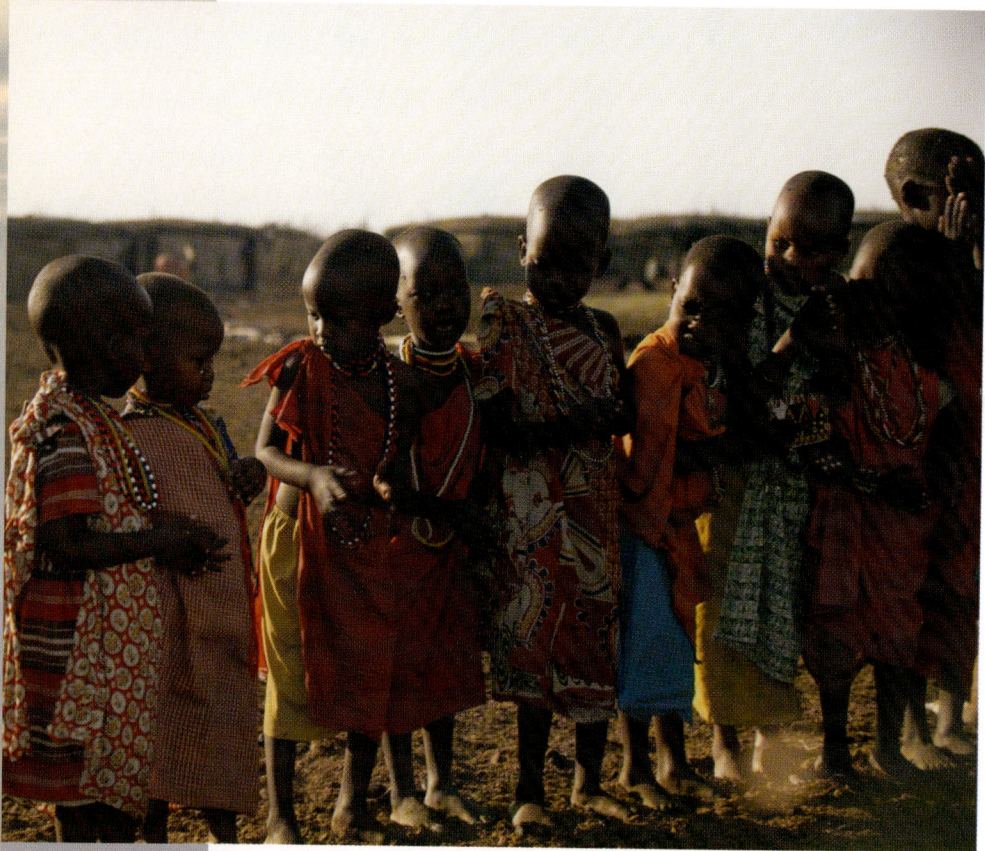

weakens the body's resistance to illness." Something as simple as a common cold can drag on because someone is undernourished and therefore does not have the physical strength to combat the invading germs.

Poor nutrition has severely hampered the treatment of individuals with HIV/AIDS in Africa. Even when antiretroviral medications are available, a lack of good nutrition may prevent the person's body from using the medicine to its best advantage.

It's not just undernutrition that can affect one's immune system, however. Research continues to show how too much food can impede the immune system. According to a report in *Nutrition and Immunity in Man*, obesity and high-fat diets can lead to an increased risk of infectious diseases. A reduction in the intake of fat can cause weight loss and, according to some researchers, decrease the risk of infectious disease by strengthening the immune system.

Researchers at the University of Illinois and Strang-Cornell Cancer Prevention Center in the United States are focusing on nutrition as a method of preventing cancer and reducing cancer deaths by strengthening the immune system. Studies are focusing on the benefits of vegetarian and low-fat diets. Though the study is ongoing, researchers believe that these dietary options would increase the body's production of disease-fighting white blood cells. Exercise also helps build the body's immune system. Athletes have their own special nutritional needs.

Nutrition and Athletes

Nutritional needs of athletes vary by type of sport, position played, and age. In general, athletes do well with a varied diet that incorporates all essential macro- and micronutrients. For most people involved in sports, gone are the days when it was believed a high-protein diet was necessary to gain muscle mass. Instead, most athletic trainers and nutritionists advocate a well-balanced diet, with a few alterations.

Did You Know?

Some athletes believe they get a boost from eating sugar or some honey just before competing. This is an old wives' tale. It takes at least thirty minutes for the sugar to enter the bloodstream. It can also cause a decrease in blood-glucose level, which can lead to fatigue.

Carbohydrates

Carbs provide the most energy for athletes, especially for those who participate in short-term, high-intensity activities such as sprinting. As with the nonathlete, complex carbs such as whole grains are recommended as opposed to sugar-based foods and drinks. According to the Olympic Training Center, a high-carb diet (up to 70 percent carbs) two to three days before an endurance event can be beneficial. A constant high-carb diet is not recommended, however, because the body will become used to using carbs, and not fatty acids, for fuel.

For events that last three hours or more, it is recommended that carbohydrate solutions—sports drinks—be consumed. However, it is important to pay attention to the drink's ingredients. They should be low in sodium. Electrolytes are not needed during competition, but they should be available afterward.

Ask the Doctor

Q: Is it always a bad thing to carry some extra weight?

No, a few pounds is not necessarily a bad thing. But excessive weight, that is, when someone can be medically termed "obese," can lead to health issues, including high blood pressure and high cholesterol. Even just a little extra weight can cause some health issues, so it is best to keep any weight gain to a minimum.

Protein

The need for protein depends on the activity. Contrary to the once-held belief that an athlete needed mega amounts of protein to build muscle, it is now known that only training builds muscle (at least naturally). According to the American Dietetic Association, most athletes will perform well with protein intake at 10 to 12 percent of total daily calories. Excess amounts of protein can lead to dehydration. The athlete's metabolic rate can increase, leading to increased use of oxygen and poor performance. Most people—including athletes—consume an adequate amount of protein, and protein supplements are ill advised.

Vitamins and Iron

Individuals who eat a diet composed of a variety of foods usually take in all of the vitamins they need. This is also true for athletes. Endurance athletes and female athletes who menstruate must take precautions that they have adequate levels of iron. Any decision to increase iron levels must be made under medical advice. Too much iron can cause constipation, diarrhea, nausea, and vomiting.

Competition Day

Contrary to what one might think, competition-day meals should not be large, heavy, or fat-laden. Most experts suggest that the meals be eaten no less than two hours before performance, and that at most, have only 1,000 calories. High-starch foods should replace high-sugar and high-fat meals. Plenty of fluids should be provided, but caffeinated products should be avoided; they can be dehydrating.

Clearly, food has a powerful effect on the body. But it isn't just our bodies that are affected by what we eat. Our mood can be affected, too.

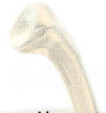

No matter what your sport, if you're an athlete, you'll have greater nutritional needs than other people.

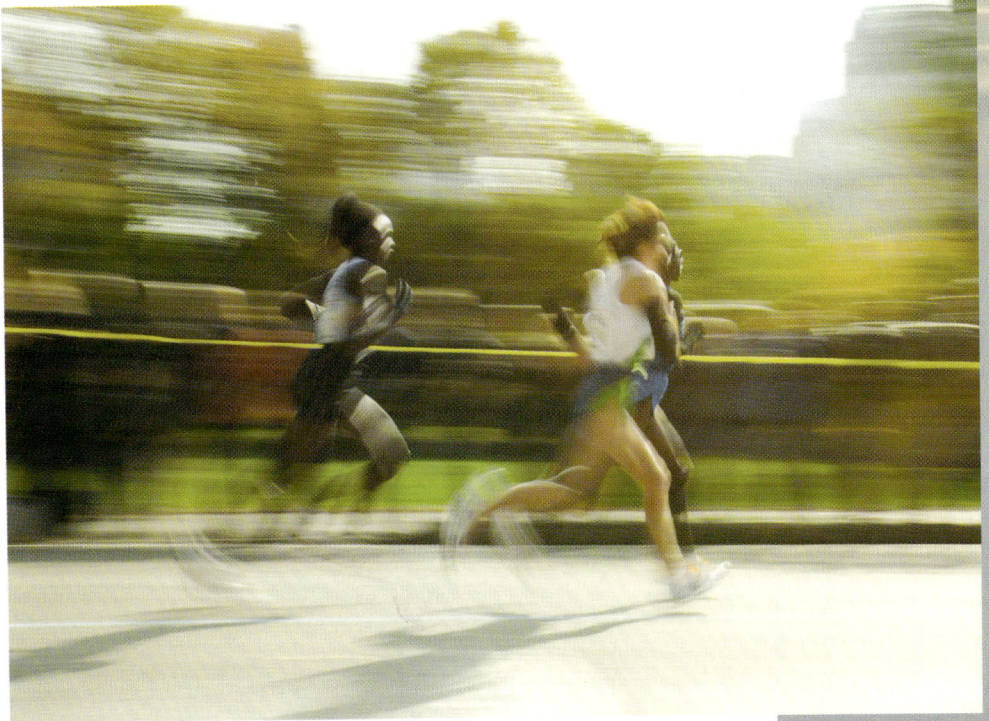

STRAIGHT FROM THE SOURCE

(From the WHO document)

Nutrition is an input to and foundation for health and development. Interaction of infection and malnutrition is well-documented. Better nutrition means stronger immune systems, less illness and better health. Healthy children learn better. Healthy people are stronger, are more productive and more able to create opportunities to gradually break the cycles of both poverty and hunger in a sustainable way. Better nutrition is a prime entry point to ending poverty and a milestone to achieving better quality of life.

Freedom from hunger and malnutrition is a basic human right and their alleviation is a fundamental prerequisite for human and national development.

WHO has traditionally focused on the vast magnitude of the many forms of nutritional deficiency, along with their associated mortality and morbidity in infants, young children and mothers. However, the world is also seeing a dramatic increase in other forms of malnutrition characterized by obesity and the long-term implications of unbalanced dietary and lifestyle practices that result in chronic diseases such as cardiovascular disease, cancer and diabetes.

All forms of malnutrition's broad spectrum are associated with significant morbidity, mortality, and economic costs, particularly in countries where both under- and overnutrition co-exist as is the case in developing countries undergoing rapid transition in nutrition and lifestyle.

What Do You Think?

- Why is freedom from hunger a basic human right?

- This document refers to "unbalanced dietary and lifestyle practices." Why is balance important to good health and nutrition?

- What do you think "overnutrition" is? Do you think it is as big a problem as malnutrition? Why or why not?

Find Out More

Go to these Web sites to discover more about nutrition and your body's functions.

Immune Central
www.immunecentral.com

Nutritional Plans for Athletes
www.chap.com.diet4.htm

Physical Inactivity: A Global Health Problem
http://www.who.int/dietphysicalactivity/factsheet_
inactivity/en/index.html

Why "Move for Health"
http://www.who.int/moveforhealth/en/

Here's what you need to know

- **There is likely a connection between the foods you crave and mood.**
- **Good nutrition is vital to the brain's communication system.**
- **Complex carbohydrates are more beneficial to your emotions than simple carbs.**

Words to Understand

An **amino acid** is an organic acid containing one or more amino groups, especially any of a group that make up proteins.

To **regenerate** is to re-form.

Insulin is a hormone secreted by the islets of Langerhans of the pancreas that regulates the blood-glucose level.

Metabolization is the process of chemical interactions that take place in living organisms that provides energy and nutrients necessary to sustain life.

4

Nutrition and Your Moods

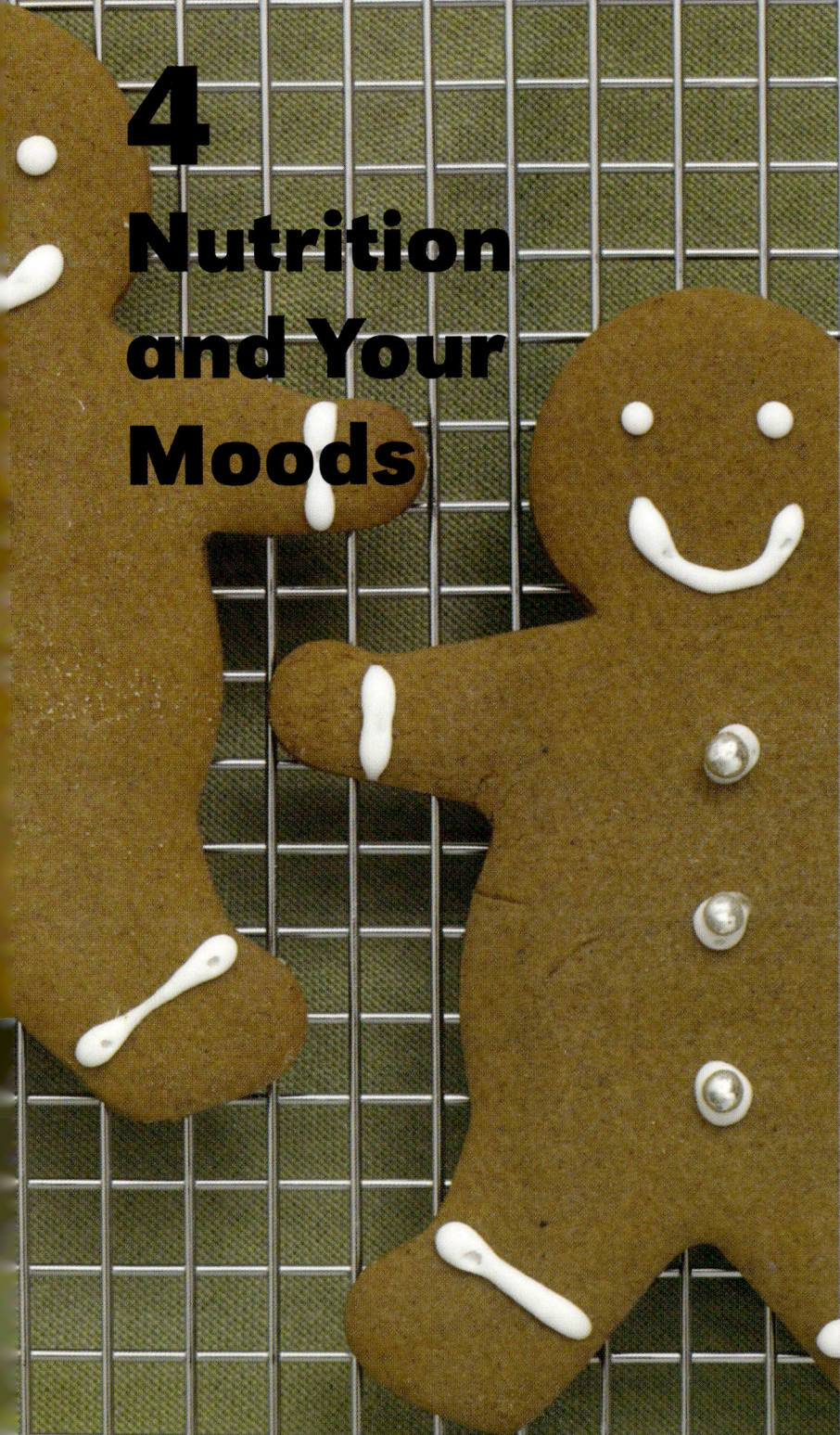

Did You Know?

The brain uses between 20 and 30 percent of a person's calorie intake at rest.

Do you know someone who wants something sugary when she feels depressed? Give her a chocolate bar, and she seems happy again. Everyone has certain foods they seem to crave when they are "down." These "comfort foods" remind of us of home or happy times. For many years, instances like these were dismissed, but researchers have begun taking a look at foods and moods, and they've found a connection.

How the Brain Communicates

The human brain is a complex messenger system. It has to be; after all, the brain is responsible for the entire body. It has to make sure that messages get from one place to another and the desired action takes place. Chemicals

Although this looks like a spindly spider, it's actually a nerve cell, which passes along messages from the brain. Neurotransmitters are what carry the messages across the tiny spaces between the nerve cells.

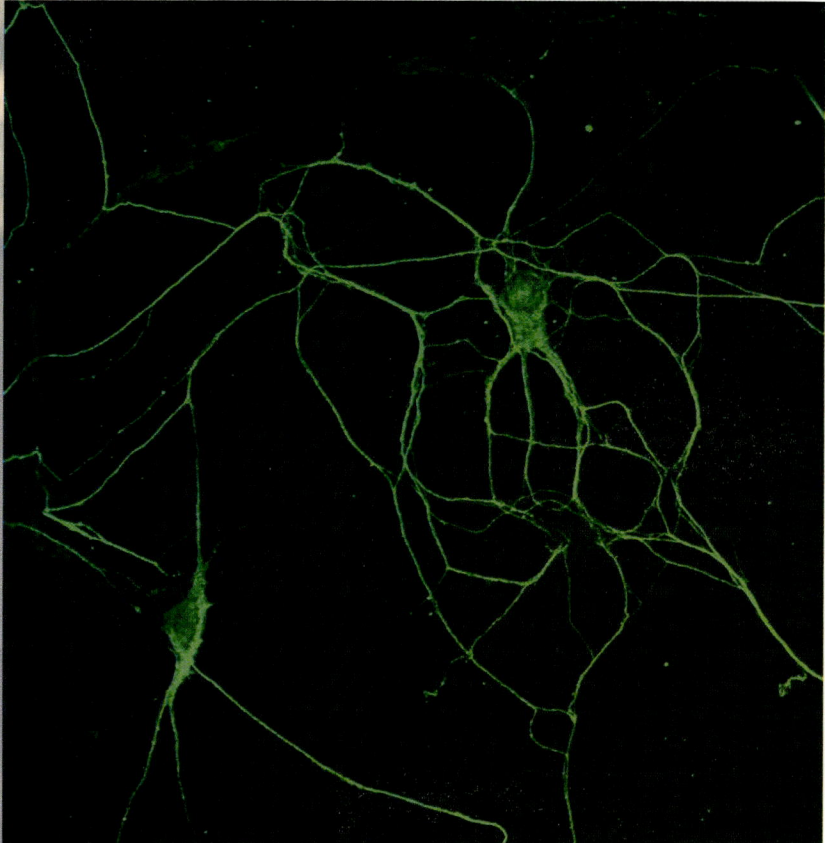

in the brain called neurotransmitters are responsible for getting electrical impulses from one nerve (or neuron) to another. Neurotransmitters also play a role in sleep patterns, thinking, and moods.

Neurotransmitters are influenced by what we take into our bodies, including food. Nutrients are basic ingredients of neurotransmitters. For example, when you eat turkey, the body takes the tryptophan, an **amino acid**, and uses it to make the neurotransmitter serotonin. Serotonin regulates sleep patterns and mood, as well as reduces anxiety.

When someone doesn't eat for a long time, the brain's communication system can become sluggish. Neurotransmitters don't have the material they need to **regenerate** or communicate effectively. As a result, individuals can become depressed, apathetic, or irritable. How they feel depends on which neurotransmitters are not being "fed." And that depends on what they do or do not eat.

Carbohydrates and Mood

Eating carbohydrates causes the release of **insulin**, a hormone. The body uses insulin to help blood glucose get into cells, where it is used as an energy source. That's why individuals may feel a rush of energy after eating a lot of carbs. But high energy levels don't last. As the insulin level increases, it allows more tryptophan to enter the brain. As mentioned earlier in this chapter, tryptophan levels are related to the level of serotonin in the brain. At first the individual feels calm, but as serotonin levels increase, the individual eventually gets sleepy

Simple carbohydrates, such as those in sugary and white flour products, break down quickly. There is a quick increase in insulin levels, which causes a quick increase in energy, but then insulin levels decrease almost as quickly. The person is hungry again for simple carbohydrates. The simple carbohydrate circle begins again.

The process takes longer with complex carbohydrates. These carbs are found in whole-grain products. Reduc-

ing the intake of simple carbs, and replacing them with complex carbs, can help produce a more steady level of serotonin available in the brain.

The carbohydrate influence on serotonin helps explain the attraction for many comfort foods. Research has shown that some people turn to carbs when they need an emotional "pick-me-up." The carbs lead to an increase in serotonin and a sense of well-being.

Proteins and Mood

Most neurotransmitters are made from amino acids. Remember from the earlier discussion that the body uses tryptophan to make serotonin. When amino acids are missing or in low supply, the body can't make the necessary levels of neurotransmitters. If the brain's supply of

What you eat and when you eat can influence your mood. If you haven't eaten all day, for instance, you may feel sad and discouraged about circumstances in your life—but things could look quite different once you've had a healthy a snack!

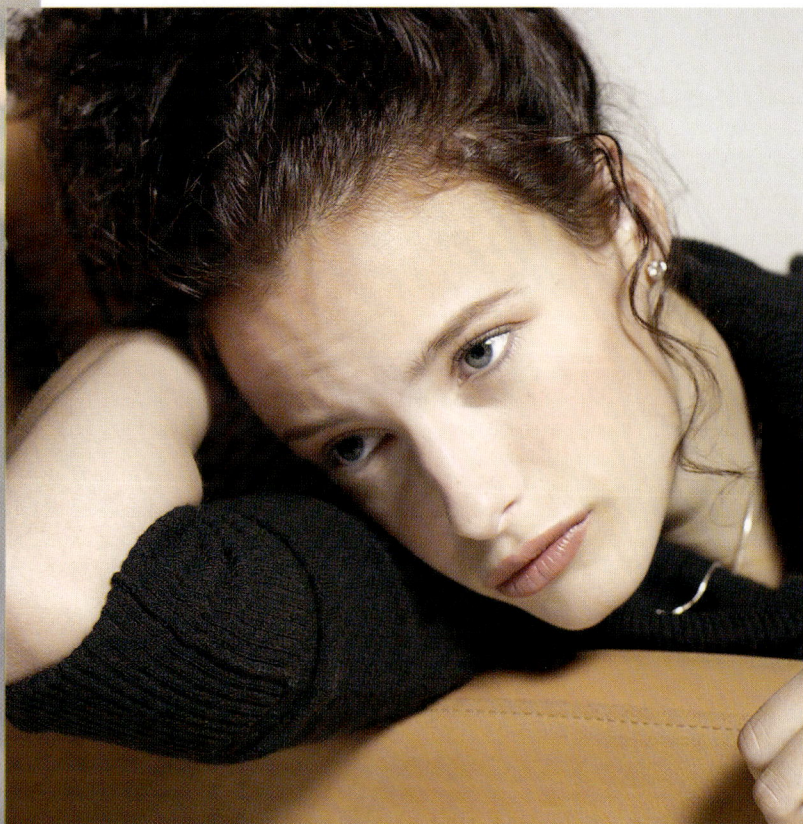

Are You an Emotional Eater?

The student health center at McMaster University (Hamilton, Ontario, Canada) offers this quiz to help you identify if you depend on food to regulate your emotions.

You've just come home after a really stressful day at school. Do you:
  A. moodily chomp through a large bag of chips or tub of ice cream and then feel even worse when you've realized what you have done?
  B. treat yourself to take-out or a couple of handfuls of cookies to cheer yourself up?
  C. eat your dinner as planned, albeit in a grumpy way?

You've just achieved a major success in your life. How do you celebrate?
  A. with unlimited chocolate/ice cream/cookies
  B. a nice meal out
  C. maybe some new clothes or an evening out, but nothing food-related

You are left alone in the room with a family-size bag of your favorite snack. Do you:
  A. break out in a cold sweat just thinking about the food, and then nervously scoff down the whole thing
  B. find it hard to resist having a bit of it
  C. eat it only if you are hungry and you're not tempted if not hungry.

How often do you think of food when you aren't eating?
  A. Food plays on my mind pretty much all the time.
  B. I do fantasize about my favorite foods sometimes.
  C. I only think about food when I work out the weekly shopping list really.

How would you rate your control over what you eat?
  A. I don't have any control. The only thing that would stop me overeating would be living three miles from the nearest grocery store with no car.
  B. Normally my diet is fairly sensible, but I do have bad days where I eat erratically without much control.
  C. I'm fully in control of what I eat.

What influences your diet the most?
  A. My mood—if I feel stressed, bored or upset, I turn to my favorite foods.
  B. A bit of everything—my mood, how hungry I am, the sort of food available.
  C. Hunger—generally, I eat when I am hungry, and when I'm full, I stop.

Turn the page for the key to your answers.

If you mostly answered A: You are an emotional eater. You may not even know what it is like to be hungry, and you may hardly even notice what food tastes like! For you, food symbolizes reward, guilt, comfort, and failure. This means that when life goes haywire so does your diet, leaving you feeling even worse. You need to learn to listen to your hunger and eat what your body actually needs.

If you mostly answered B: You are a variable eater. Most of the time, you have a fairly balanced attitude to food, but on a bad day, you lose that. Many people fall into this category, and the odd bad day when you eat too much chocolate cake probably won't do too much harm. But if your attitude to food is making you feel bad, or making it hard to maintain a healthy weight, then you need to find alternative ways of coping with stress.

Mostly answered C: You are a functional eater. You enjoy your meals, but what you eat has little to do with your mood. In our society, where food is available everywhere, your cool-headed attitude to food should help you to maintain a healthy body weight.

a neurotransmitter is low, this can manifest in a change in mood or behavior. People with a low serotonin level, for example, may be sad, perhaps even depressed. Some research has shown a connection between low levels of serotonin and aggressive behavior.

Fats and Mood

The biological connection between fat intake and mood is not as clear-cut as the relationship between carbohydrates, proteins, and mood. Researchers have studied the influence of omega-3 fatty acids on individuals with bipolar and stress disorders. Preliminary findings have shown that there may be a benefit, but more studies are needed.

Other studies are looking into the effect of fat on mood changes and aggressive behavior. Some research has found that reducing fat levels can actually lower the level of serotonin available in the brain. This often leads to mood swings and aggressive behavior. Before any recommendations are made concerning fat and mood, more studies need to be done.

Vitamins and Moods

Vitamins, especially the B family of vitamins, also play a role in moods. Studies conducted by the Human Nutrition Research Center of the U.S. Department of Agriculture have found that a lack of B vitamins can lead to "impaired memory and higher levels of anxiety, confusion, irritability, and depression."

Thiamin is tied to the **metabolization** of glucose, which is the primary source of energy for the brain. It is also used to make many of the brain's neurotransmitters.

B_{12} helps maintain the myelin layer, which covers the nerve cells in the brain. If this protective covering is damaged or inadequate, the nerve itself can be damaged. Such damage can lead to dementia. Most people who eat a well-balanced diet get enough B_{12}. However, individuals who eat a strict vegan diet—no meat or dairy products—may need to take a supplement, because the vitamin is found only in animal products.

Niacin is a factor in the release of energy from carbs, proteins, and fats. If the body lacks niacin, sleep disorders, memory loss, and emotional instability can result. Pellagra, a severe form of niacin deficiency, can lead to psychosis or delirium. In the United States, niacin is found in meat, fish, peanuts, asparagus, and enriched grains. While niacin deficiency was once a problem in the United States, as diets have improved, it has become increasingly rare. It is still a problem in India, China, and some developing countries.

Though nutrition plays a role in moods, it is unlikely that a nutritional disorder is completely responsible for a mood disorder. It is something to consider during diagnosis and treatment, however. Nutrition affects every part of the body, including the brain.

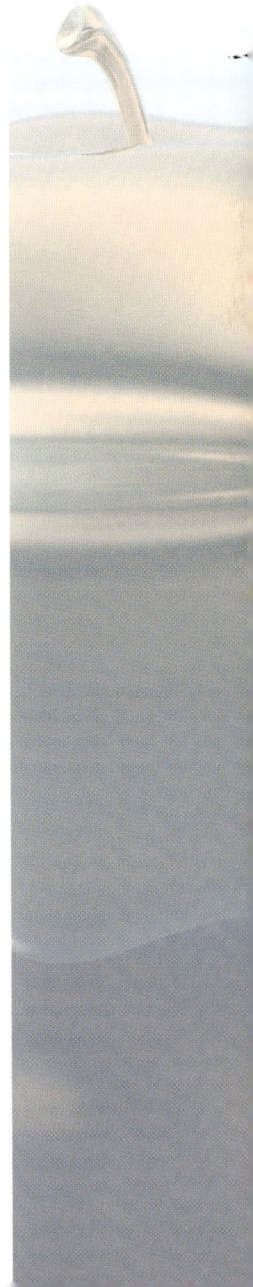

STRAIGHT FROM THE SOURCE

(From the National Institutes of Health Web site document, Brain Serotonin, Carbohydrate-Craving, Obesity, and Depression)

Serotonin and Food

Serotonin-releasing brain neurons are unique in that the amount of neurotransmitter they release is normally controlled by food intake: Carbohydrate consumption—acting via insulin secretion and the "plasma tryptophan ratio"—increases serotonin release; protein intake lacks this effect. This ability of neurons to couple neuronal signaling properties to food consumption is a link in the feedback mechanism that normally keeps carbohydrate and protein intakes more or less constant. However, serotonin release is also involved in such functions as sleep onset, pain sensitivity, blood pressure regulation, and control of the mood. Hence many patients learn to overeat carbohydrates (particularly snack foods, like potato chips or pastries, which are rich in carbohydrates and fats) to make themselves feel better. This tendency to use certain foods as though they were drugs is a frequent cause of weight gain, and can also be seen in patients who become fat when exposed to stress, or in women with premenstrual syndrome, or in patients with "winter depression," or in people who are attempting to give up smoking.

Parkdale Secondary School

What Do You Think?

- What foods make you feel better?

- What things can someone do who is trying to stop smoking—besides eat?

- In what ways do people use food as though it was a drug?

Find Out More

Go to these Web sites to find out more about the connection between food and mood.

Food and Mood
www.dbsalliance.org/pdfs/foodmoode2.pdf

Food and Your Mood
www.realbuzz.com/en-gb/food_and_your_mood/
index?pageID=1329

Garibaldi Secondary School
24789 Dewdney Trunk Road
Maple Ridge, B.C.
V4R 1X2

Here's what you need to know

- **Healthy neurotransmitters are essential to the brain's communication system.**
- **Glucose is the brain's most important necessity.**
- **The brain uses carbohydrates and fats and proteins to function most efficiently.**
- **Omega-3 fatty acids play an important role in overall good health.**

Words to Understand

Homocysteines are amino acids that can be harmful and lead to heart disease in large quantities.

Norepinephrine is a neurotransmitter.

An **axon** is an extension of a nerve cell, similar in shape to a thread, that transmits impulses outward from the cell body.

An **antioxidant** is any substance that inhibits the destructive effects of oxidation.

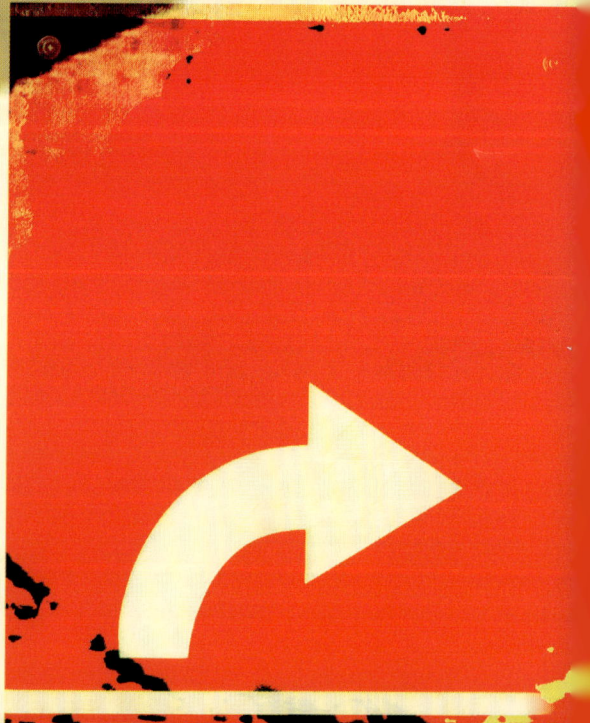

5

Nutrition and Your Brain

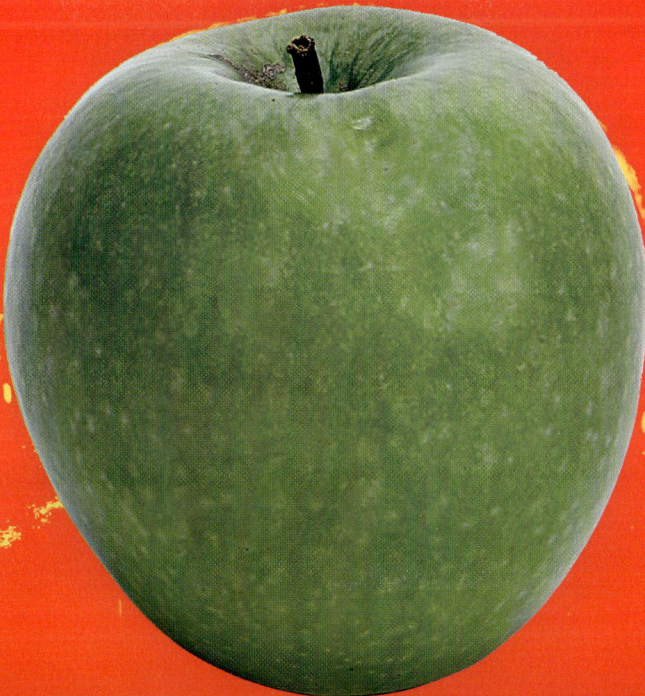

Though it weighs only about three pounds, the human brain is command central for the entire body. Like the rest of the body, the brain needs to be fed—and not just with information. Good nutrition is necessary for the brain to function at its optimum, so it can tell the rest of the body what to do.

Breakfast is the meal that gives your body fuel for the day. A healthy breakfast includes whole grains, some kind of protein (whether milk or meat), and fruit.

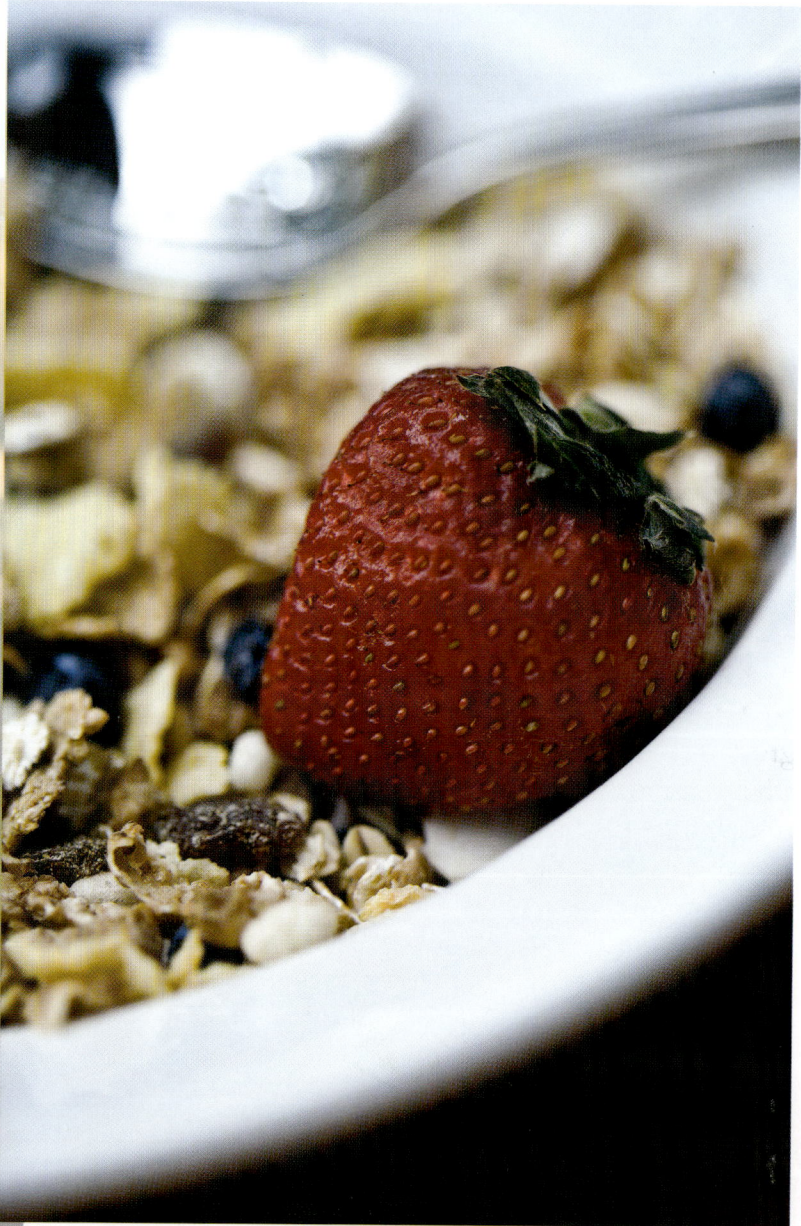

What the Brain Needs

As discussed in the previous chapter, the brain uses neurotransmitters to send messages to all parts of the body. The "recipe" for making these neurotransmitters includes ingredients from food. For example, the body uses tyrosine, found in milk, meat, fish, and legumes, to make norepinephrine, which affects alertness. When the diet is missing certain key elements, it may not be possible for the brain to build all of the neurotransmitters it needs for its message system. The brain uses carbohydrates, fats, and proteins to function most efficiently.

Carbohydrates

The brain has very specific dietary needs. Its most important requirement is glucose. The body converts carbohydrates (and some other foods) into glucose. There is a popular American saying, "Breakfast is the most important meal of the day." Well, according to many scientific studies, this saying is right on target. For the brain to operate at its best throughout the day, it needs a steady supply of glucose, starting with a healthy breakfast.

Keep in mind, though, that there are differences between carbohydrates. Carbohydrates are found in bread, pasta, rice, fruit, and refined sugars. The body benefits most from complex carbohydrates. In the case of grains, these would be in foods made of whole wheat and whole grains. As the flour and grain becomes more processed, many of the natural characteristics are removed and things are added, such as solid fat and sugar. The food's healthy benefits to the body, including the brain, decrease. Though eating a piece of toast made of white bread immediately satisfies one's hunger, its effects wear off more quickly than if the person had eaten whole-wheat toast. Not only does this affect alertness, memory, and other things necessary for school and work performance, choosing the wrong kind of carbohydrates can lead to overeating and obesity.

Did You Know?

The FAO recommends that at least 55% of an individual's total daily diet should come from a variety of carbohydrates, especially whole-grain cereals, root vegetables, and fruits.

Did You Know?

Some cities are banning the use of trans fats in restaurant cooking.

Did You Know?

You know how great it is to have a nice mug of hot chocolate on a cold winter day? Well, studies have shown that you're doing your brain a favor, too. A Cornell University chemist has discovered that two tablespoons of pure cocoa—not the chocolate drink mix—have more antioxidants than red wine, green tea, or black tea.

Fats and Proteins

Looking at the media attention surrounding fats, and at times proteins, might give one the idea that they are threatening the existence of the entire human species. That's not quite accurate. When it comes to the brain, it is actually very wrong. When protein-rich foods and fats are digested, amino acids and fatty acids result. Without the proper amount of these substances, the nervous system cannot function properly.

The brain uses the by-products of proteins and fats to make myelin. Myelin, a white substance that surrounds many axons, is made of approximately 80 percent fat and 20 percent protein. It increases the speed at which impulses travel along the **axon**, as well as helps prevent electrical current from leaving the axon.

Like carbohydrates, the brain functions best with certain proteins, and especially certain fats. Two of the most important fats for the brain are omego-3 fatty acid and n-6 fatty acid. The fatty acids are found in such foodstuffs as fatty fish and flax. They are also found in milk and eggs, but in higher quantities in organic milk and eggs from free-range chickens fed a diet high in greens and insects rather than corn.

A study reported in the *Journal of Neuroscience* showed that these fatty acids may have a role in memory retention. Some research has shown that a diet lacking in omega-3 and n-6 fatty acids may be a factor in learning disabilities and problems with motor coordination.

Is There Such a Thing as a "Smart Food"?

Wouldn't it be nice if we could eat, oh, say a banana, and find ourselves smarter than we had been before the banana? That's probably not going to happen—at least not anytime soon and probably not without some genetic "tweaking" of the banana. But that *doesn't* mean there might not be a connection between what we eat and our intelligence. We've already seen how foods affect some aspects of the brain.

Researchers have been looking for a connection between food and intelligence for many years. And while they haven't found a food that will make someone instantly smarter, they have found dietary ways to improve brain functioning. Scientists for the Agricultural Research Service have found a connection between *antioxidant*-rich foods, such as spinach and strawberries, and brain function. In another study, rats equivalent in age to sixty-three human years were fed a diet high in spinach and strawberry extracts. When tested eight weeks later, age-related cognitive losses had been reversed. Those fed blueberry extract had even better results. Wild blueberries have also been found to improve memory and motor skills, including coordination.

Ask the Doctor

Q: Does it make a difference whether I use margarine or vegetable oil?

Many margarines contain trans fats, which research has shown to be harmful over time. Vegetable oils do not contain trans fats and are not as harmful. However, that doesn't mean you can use as much as you want. Moderation is the key in using both vegetable oil and margarine.

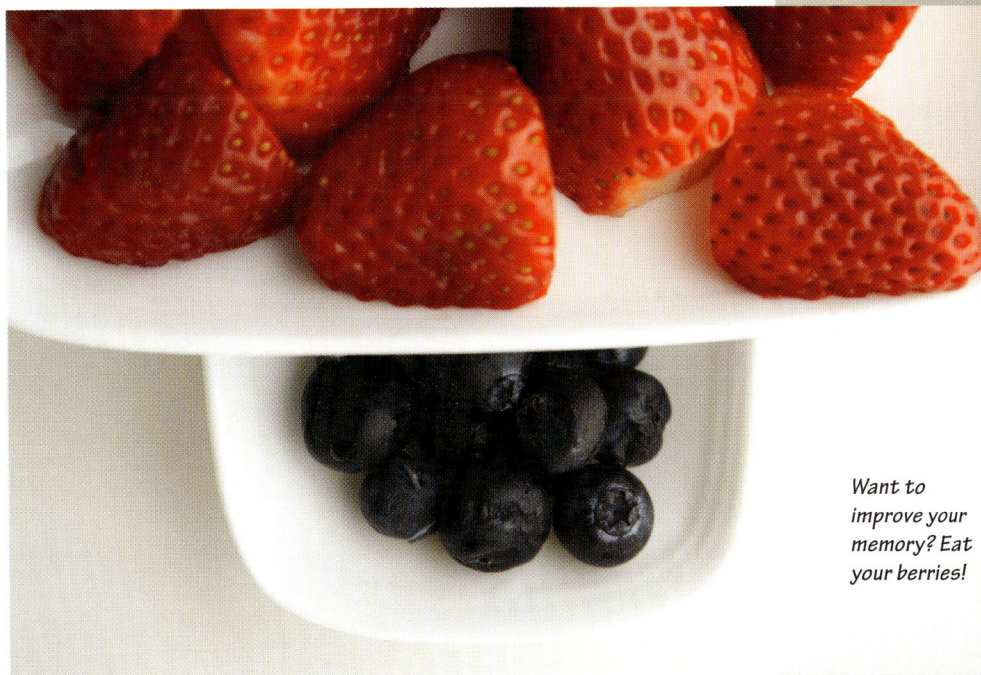

Want to improve your memory? Eat your berries!

Dark, leafy greens, such as collard greens and swiss chard have been shown to slow cognitive decline that is associated with Alzheimer's disease. It is believed that the folate and B_{12} found in these greens help break down

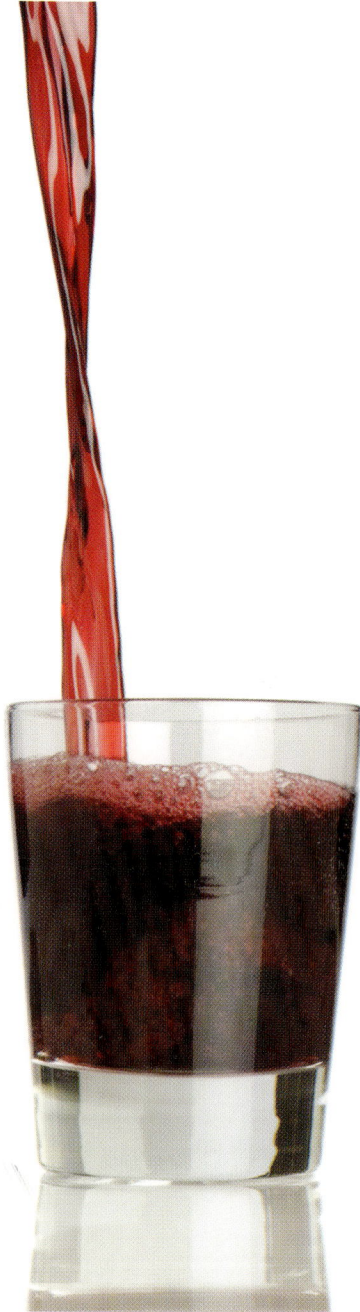

The benefits of grape juice on the brain come from flavonoids. Natural antioxidants, flavonoids mop up the harmful free radicals generated when cells burn oxygen for energy.

the **homocysteines**. Most research shows a relationship between high levels of homocysteines and Alzheimer's. And Popeye isn't the only one to benefit from spinach. Switch the iceberg (head) lettuce for spinach, and your salad will have three times the amount of folate.

As discussed earlier in the chapter, fatty fish (including salmon, sardines, and herring) contain large amounts of the beneficial omega-3 fatty acids, which help neurotransmitters communicate with each other. According to a study conducted by the Rush Institute for Healthy Aging, people who eat just one fish meal per week are less likely to develop Alzheimer's disease.

Concord grape juice can improve short-term memory and motor skills. According to studies conducted by the Human Nutrition Research Center on Aging, concord grape juice has the highest antioxidant level of any fruit or vegetable tested thus far.

No matter how much you learn about the importance of good nutrition, some factors make having a healthy diet difficult. Some are within your control, but others may not be.

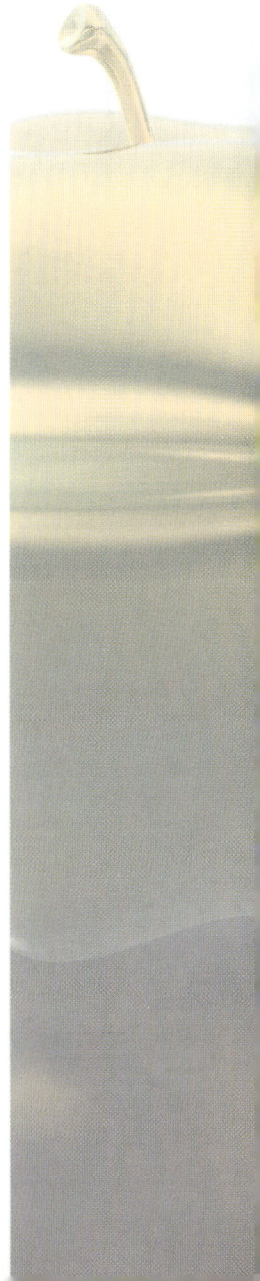

STRAIGHT FROM THE SOURCE

(From the U.S. Food and Agriculture Organization document, Fish Is Food for the Brain as Well as Good Protein.)

Fish and the Brain

Fish is a food of excellent nutritional value, providing high quality protein and a wide variety of vitamins and minerals, including vitamins A and D, phosphorus, magnesium, selenium, and iodine in marine fish. Its protein—like that of meat—is easily digestible and favourably complements dietary protein provided by cereals and legumes that are typically consumed in many developing countries.

Experts agree that, even in small quantities, fish can have a significant positive impact in improving the quality of dietary protein by complementing the essential amino acids that are often present in low quantities in vegetable-based diets.

But recent research shows that fish is much more than just an alternative source of animal protein. Fish oils in fatty fish are the richest source of a type of fat that is vital to normal brain development in unborn babies and infants. Without adequate amounts of these fatty acids, normal brain development does not take place.

What Do You Think?

• How can people be encouraged to eat more fish?

• How can fish be used to combat food shortages?

• What can people do to get more fish into their diets if they live where fishing has been limited due to water contamination?

Find Out More

Go to these Web sites to find out more about nutrition and your brain:

The Human Brain
222.fi.edu/learn/brain/diet.html

What Is Good Brain Food?
psychologytoday.com/articles/pto-20031028-000010.html

Here's what you need to know

- **Poverty is one of the biggest impediments to good nutrition worldwide.**
- **Food allergies are on the rise in North America, Europe, Japan, and Australia.**
- **Though there is evidence that the "diet mentality" is lessening, it continues to be a problem, leading many to develop eating disorders.**

Words to Understand

Anaphylactic means relating to or caused by extreme sensitivity to a substance.

Body Mass Index (BMI) is a measure of your weight divided by the square of your height. It provides a rough estimate of your percentage of body fat.

Anorexia is an eating disorder characterized by an extreme fear of becoming overweight, leading to extreme dieting.

Bulimia is an eating disorder in which periods of overeating are followed by undereating, the use of laxatives, or self-induced vomiting.

Rickets is a disease usually caused by a lack of vitamin D that softens bones.

Scurvy is a disease caused by not eating enough vitamin C.

68

6

Good Nutrition's Enemies

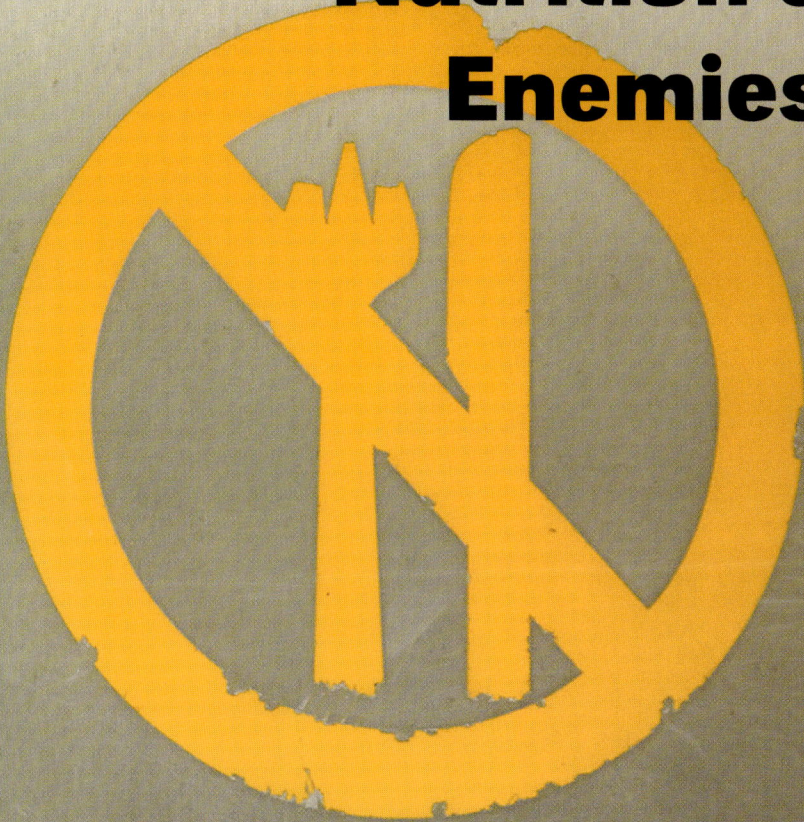

People who live in poverty—whether in one of the world's developed nations, like this man, or in one of the developing nations—have fewer food resources. This means that many of them experience malnutrition and undernutrition.

Most people want to be healthy. Some are even willing to work at it. But when it comes to good nutrition, that isn't always enough. For some people, there are factors that work against getting good nutrition. Some they can control; others they can't.

Poverty

One of the biggest impediments to good nutrition is poverty. According to the World Health Organization, almost 30 percent of all people in the world suffer from at least one form of malnutrition.

Poverty's effect on malnutrition in third-world and developing countries also influences how they fight dis-

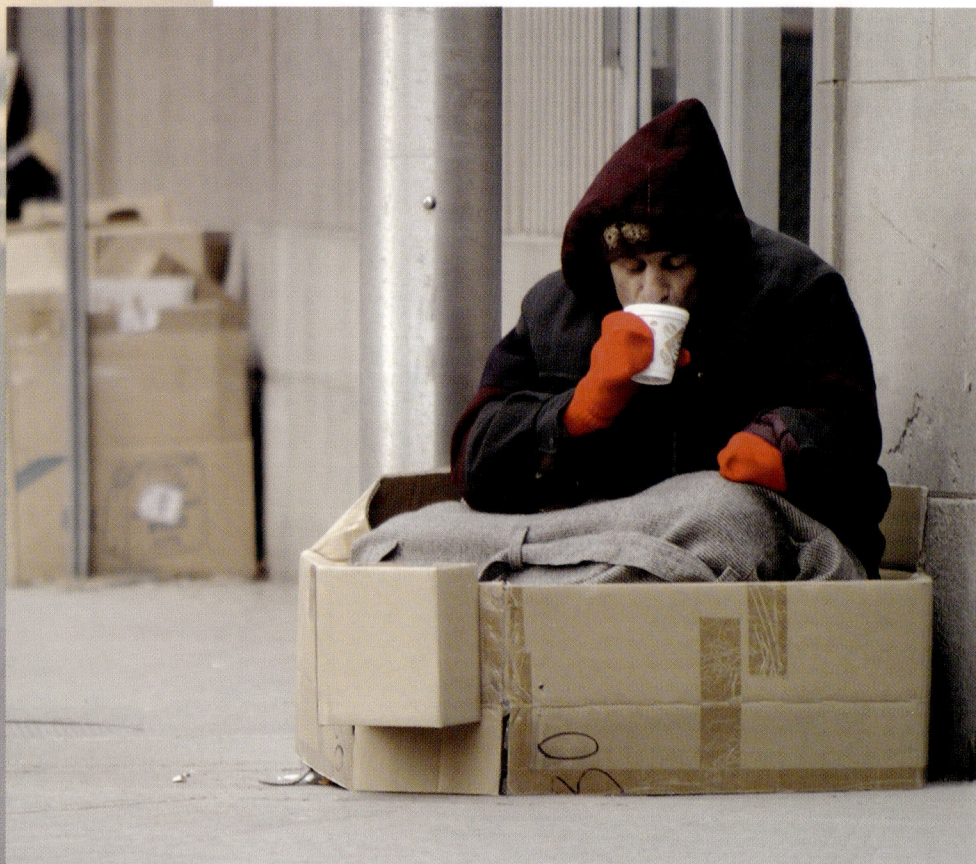

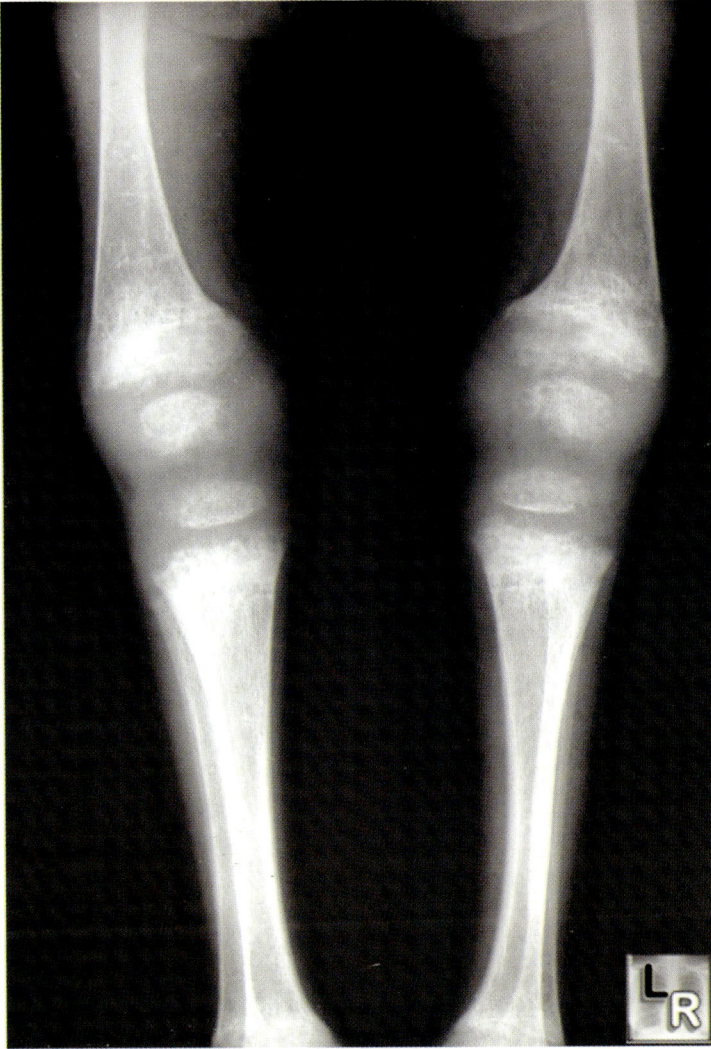

This X-ray shows the leg bones of a child with rickets, a softening of the bones that can lead to fractures and the bow-legged appearance shown here. Rickets is among the most frequent childhood diseases in many developing countries. The most common cause is a vitamin D deficiency, but not enough calcium in the diet can also lead to rickets. Although rickets can occur in adults, the majority of cases occur in children suffering from the severe malnutrition of starvation and famine during the early years of their lives.

ease. Some diseases, such as rickets and scurvy, are common among people who are undernourished. Malnutrition can make it difficult to fight diseases such as HIV/AIDS. This means that diseases can be spread, infecting an even larger proportion of the population. And people who are very ill may not be able to work to support their families, meaning that malnutrition goes on to affect another generation.

Poverty is not limited to developing countries. In prosperous countries as well, not everyone gets the food they

Did You Know?

According to the WHO, approximately 60 percent of the 10.9 million deaths of children under age five in developing countries are related to malnutrition.

need. Lack of income influences nutritional decisions all around the world. For example, according to the Bread for the World Institute, in 2001, there were approximately 33 million children in the United States who did not know when they would get their next meal. Government and private-sector programs, including the school lunch program, can step in to help individuals get the assistance they need. In the meantime, these individuals may be lacking in important nutrients.

Fast Food

Every day we make decisions about food. One of those decisions might be to eat at a fast-food restaurant. After all, it's fast, convenient, and relatively inexpensive. It might seem counterintuitive, but it can be less expensive to stop

Soft drinks and fast foods have become a part of many teenagers' lifestyles. They're quick and convenient sources of calories. Unfortunately, they offer few nutrients.

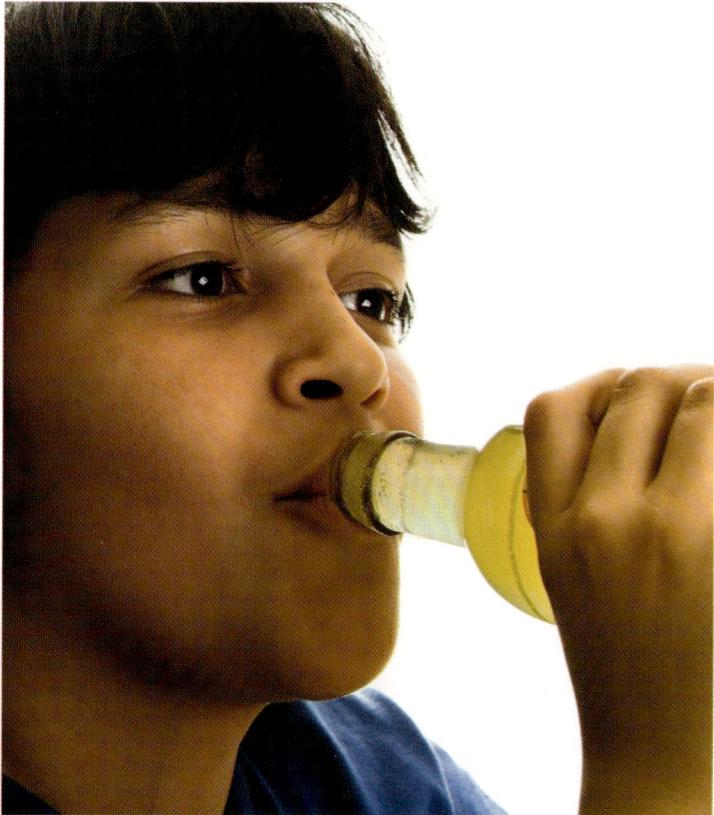

at a fast-food restaurant than to cook at home, which makes it particularly attractive to people with a low income. In many locations, it is cheaper to buy a complete meal than to go to a supermarket and buy fresh ingredients to make one, especially with the promotions the restaurants give to stay one step ahead of their competitors. And with the busy schedules many people juggle, going to a fast-food restaurant may seem to be the only way to fit everything into a day. So, healthy, fresh fruits and vegetables are passed over in favor of a fast-food meal. Though people may save time and money in the short term, over time the decision can be costly for their health. Even fast-food options listed as "healthy" may have hidden fats and calories. These add up and can lead to obesity and the problems associated with being overweight.

Disease/Food Allergies

Some individuals have medical conditions that make it difficult to receive some of the nutrients they need. These include:

- celiac disease: a sensitivity to gluten
- lactose intolerance: a low level or absence of the enzyme lactase, which is needed to digest milk sugar
- pernicious anemia: individuals are unable to absorb B_{12}

    In many cases, alternative foods are available or medication can be given to counter the nutritional deficits caused by these conditions.

    According to the Food and Agriculture Organization, there is a growing problem of food allergies in North America, Europe, and Australia, especially among infants

Ask the Doctor

Ask the Doctor
Q: Do I have to give up fast food to be healthy?

No, you don't have to give it up entirely, but it shouldn't be an everyday thing. And when you're there, learn to make smart food choices. Instead of a hamburger, order a chicken sandwich, but make sure the chicken is grilled or broiled rather than fried. Don't order the largest fries or soft drink on the menu. And, if you can substitute fruit for fries, do so.

Did You Know?

Over 170 foods have been documented as causing food allergies.

and young children. Some of the more prevalent allergies are to:

• nuts, especially peanuts
• eggs
• high-acid foods and fruits such as oranges and tomatoes
• shellfish

Allergic reactions can range from a slight rash to anaphylactic shock. Again, for individuals with food allergies, there are usually other foods that can provide the nutrients. In some cases, supplements may be necessary.

Peanut allergies are becoming increasingly common. Some people are so allergic that they may have a reaction if they eat food that was prepared in the same factory with other foods that contain peanuts—or if they even inhale a few drops from an aerosol cooking spray containing peanut oil.

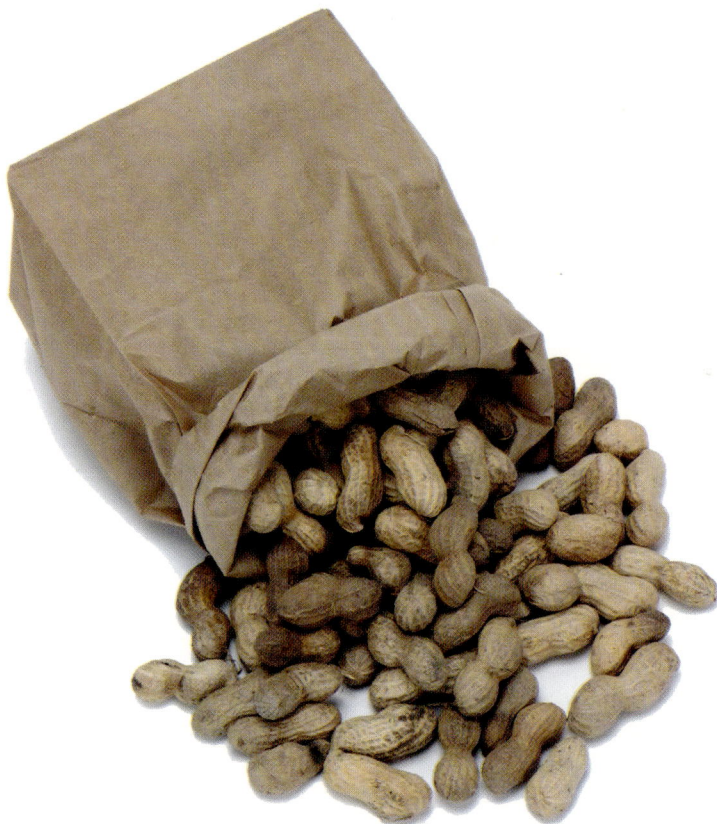

Real People

Thirteen-year-old Jesse Milliner is allergic to most nuts, but especially peanuts. When he had his first allergic reaction, his mom knew what to do, since his older brother, Jeremy, has a nut allergy—but not to peanuts. The boys' reactions can range from a tingly mouth to swelling of the lips and throat. Their parents always make sure to have an Epi-pen handy in case of severe emergencies. Some people with nut allergies cannot even touch one without having a reaction. Jesse and Jeremy are "lucky"; they have to consume nuts to have a reaction.

It's not always easy for Jesse and Jeremy, or their parents, to know if something contains nuts. Naomi, their mother, spends a lot of time reading labels. And because peanut butter is a popular school lunch item, Jesse's school has a special table where students who are allergic to nuts can sit and eat without worrying about exposure.

Bad Eating Habits

Sometimes nutrition suffers simply because we get into bad eating habits. We take the "easy way out" and stop at a fast-food restaurant or pick up something "ready-made" from a street vendor. Once in a while, that's usually not a problem, but when it becomes a habit, nutrition can suffer. Many of these items have high fat and sodium contents. In most cases, the fats used in such products are not the healthier poly- and monounsaturated fats. Instead, manufacturers use saturated fats and trans fats.

Another habit individuals sometimes fall into is eating the same thing over and over again. Or perhaps they eat

The UK's Food Standards Agency did a survey of UK teens. Here are the results:

- more than 50% said they had been on a diet at least once and 10% admitted to always being on a diet. "To look thin" was one of their main reasons for changing your diets (more important than having energy for exercise).
- 15% would even consider taking laxatives or making themselves sick to lose weight .
- 25% say they try to eat as little as possible.
- 42% regularly skip breakfast.
- Nearly 50% drink soda every day.
- 10% eat fast food at least once a day.
- 83% aren't eating the recommended five portions of fruit and vegetables a day.

things from only one or two food groups. Remember that healthy nutrition requires eating a variety of foods.

Breaking bad habits is not easy. After all, you don't start a habit in just one day; you can't expect to break one that quickly. But the good news is that you *can* break them. It takes time and effort.

The "Diet" Mentality

Young women around the world dream of becoming supermodels—yet very few attain the dream. The truth is, it is probably healthier for them if they are unsuccessful. In 2006, at a fashion show in Madrid, Spain, models were not allowed to walk unless they had a Body Mass Index (BMI) of at least 18. Many models failed the test, meaning their body weights were so low they were unhealthy. In the modeling world, Emme and Mia Tyler are called "plus-size" models, even though they are closer in size to an average woman than better-known models such as Kate Moss and Gisele Bündchen.

Many people, especially—though not exclusively—girls, have fallen prey to the desire to be ultrathin. This has led to an explosion in the number of people with anorexia, bulimia, and other eating disorders. The road back to good health can be long and hard. For some, such as singer Karen Carpenter, it comes too late. The effects of eating disorders on the body can be fatal.

There is some evidence that the "thinner is better" mentality has begun to shift toward a more moderate, healthier outlook. Singer/actress Queen Latifah has

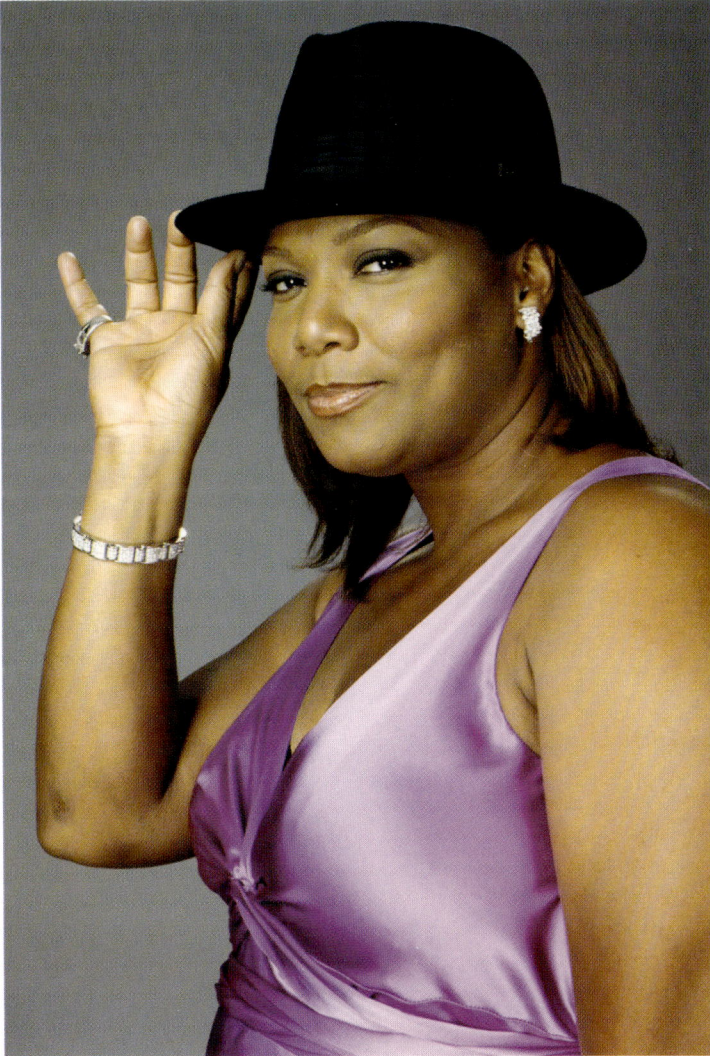

Queen Latifah is showing the world that you don't have to be skin and bones to be beautiful.

Jennifer Lopez doesn't try to conform to the pencil-thin body type so popular among actresses and models. She's proud of her body.

become the spokesperson for the weight-loss company Jenny Craig. Her goal, she clearly states, is to get to a healthier weight—not to get skinny. Actress/author Jamie Lee Curtis has spoken out against the pressure to be thin. Pink has extolled the virtues of being true to who you are in her songs. Singer/actress Jennifer Lopez takes pride in her curvy body. And don't forget, singer/actress Jennifer Hudson didn't hide her figure when she picked up an Oscar® for her performance in *Dreamgirls*.

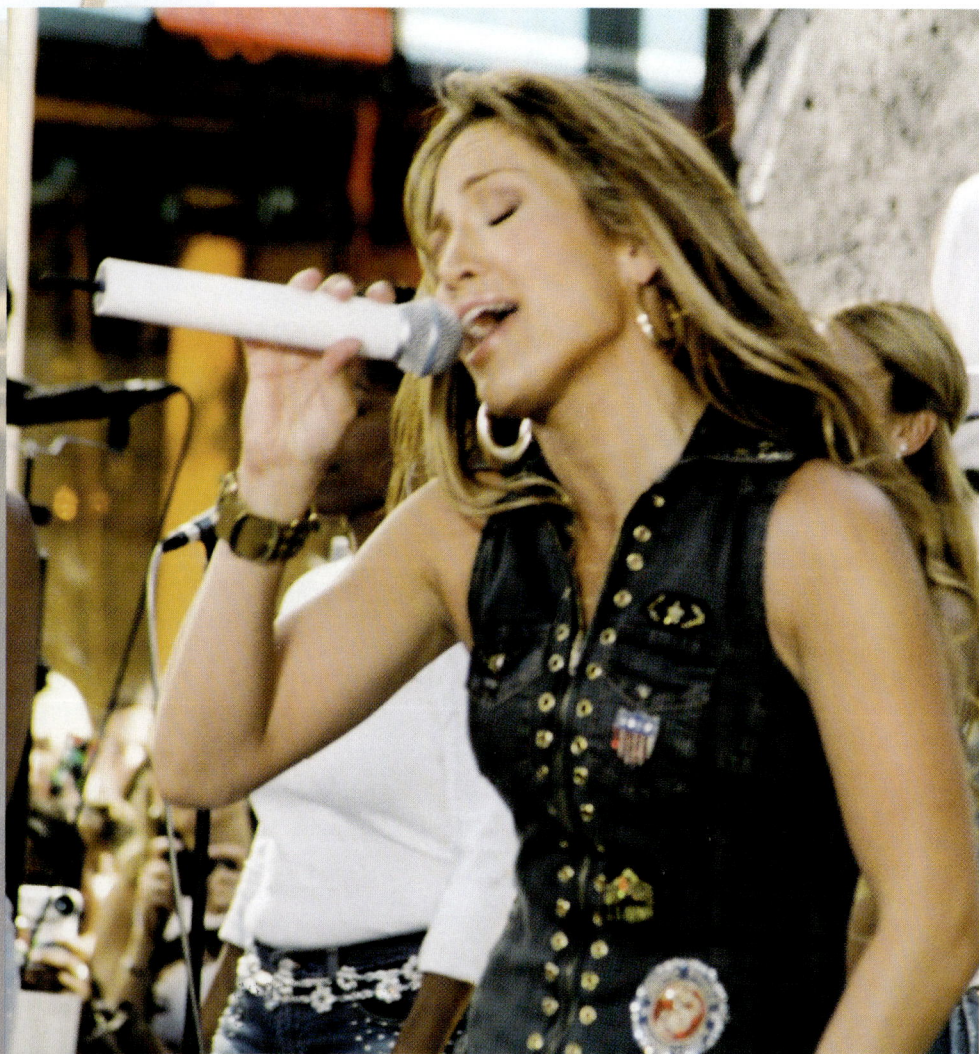

"Ordinary" people can also see a change when they go shopping for clothes. The selection of clothes above size 6 has grown.

It's important to realize that just as too thin can be bad, so can being too heavy. Obesity has become a major global health concern.

The long-term effects of obesity can be similar to some that characterize malnutrition. Studies have shown that the immune system can be compromised by excessive weight. And, of course, the incidence of heart disease, high blood pressure, and diabetes dramatically increases along with weight. Each person benefits by finding the weight at which she is the healthiest.

Garibaldi Secondary School
24789 Dewdney Trunk Road
Maple Ridge, B.C.
V4R 1X2

STRAIGHT FROM THE SOURCE

(From the WHO document, Nutrition for Health and Development)

Controlling the Global Obesity Epidemic

At the other end of the malnutrition scale, obesity is one of today's most blatantly visible—yet most neglected—public health problems. Paradoxically coexisting with undernutrition, an escalating global epidemic of overweight and obesity—"globesity"—is taking over many parts of the world. If immediate action is not taken, millions will suffer from an array of serious health disorders.

Obesity is a complex condition, one with serious social and psychological dimensions, that affects virtually all age and socioeconomic groups and threatens to overwhelm both developed and developing countries. In 1995, there were an estimated 200 million obese adults worldwide and another 18 million under-five children classified as overweight. As of 2000, the number of obese adults has increased to over 300 million. Contrary to conventional wisdom, the obesity epidemic is not restricted to industrialized societies; in developing countries, it is estimated that over 115 million people suffer from obesity-related problems.

Generally, although men may have higher rates of overweight, women have higher rates of obesity. For both, obesity poses a major risk for serious diet-related noncommunicable diseases, including diabetes mellitus, cardiovascular disease, hypertension and stroke, and certain forms of cancer. Its health consequences range from increased risk of premature death to serious chronic conditions that reduce the overall quality of life.

The response: making healthy choices easy choices

WHO began sounding the alarm in the 1990s, spearheading a series of expert and technical consultations. Public awareness campaigns were also initiated to sensitize policy-makers, private sector partners, medical professionals and the public at large. Aware that obesity is predominantly a "social and environmental disease", WHO is helping to develop strategies that will make healthy choices easier to make. In collaboration with the University of Sydney (Australia), WHO is calculating the worldwide economic impact of overweight and obesity. It is also working with the University of Auckland (New Zealand) to analyse the impact that globalization and rapid socioeconomic transition have on nutrition and to identify the main political, socioeconomic, cultural and physical factors which promote obesogenic environments.

What Do You Think?

- Why do you think an obesity problem is going on in the world at the same time an undernourishment problem is?

- Why do you think obesity is a "social and environmental disease"? What do you think this means?

- Why do think there is a worldwide economic impact from obesity?

- Using the context, what do you think "obesogenic" means?

Find Out More

Check out these Web sites to find out more about access to good nutrition around the world:

Bread for the World
www.bread.org

CommonDreams
www.commondreams.org

Here's what you need to know

Here's What You Need to Know
- **You need to eat a variety of foods.**
- **Slow down and you'll eat less.**
- **Physical activity is also part of good health.**

Words to Understand

Moderation means just the right amount, neither too much nor too little.

A **pit stop** is literally a racers' stop at a pit for refueling or service during an automobile race. It's fast, frantic, and definitely not relaxed.

Overtaxed means carrying a heavy burden or strain that's more than can be easily endured.

7
Food for Thought

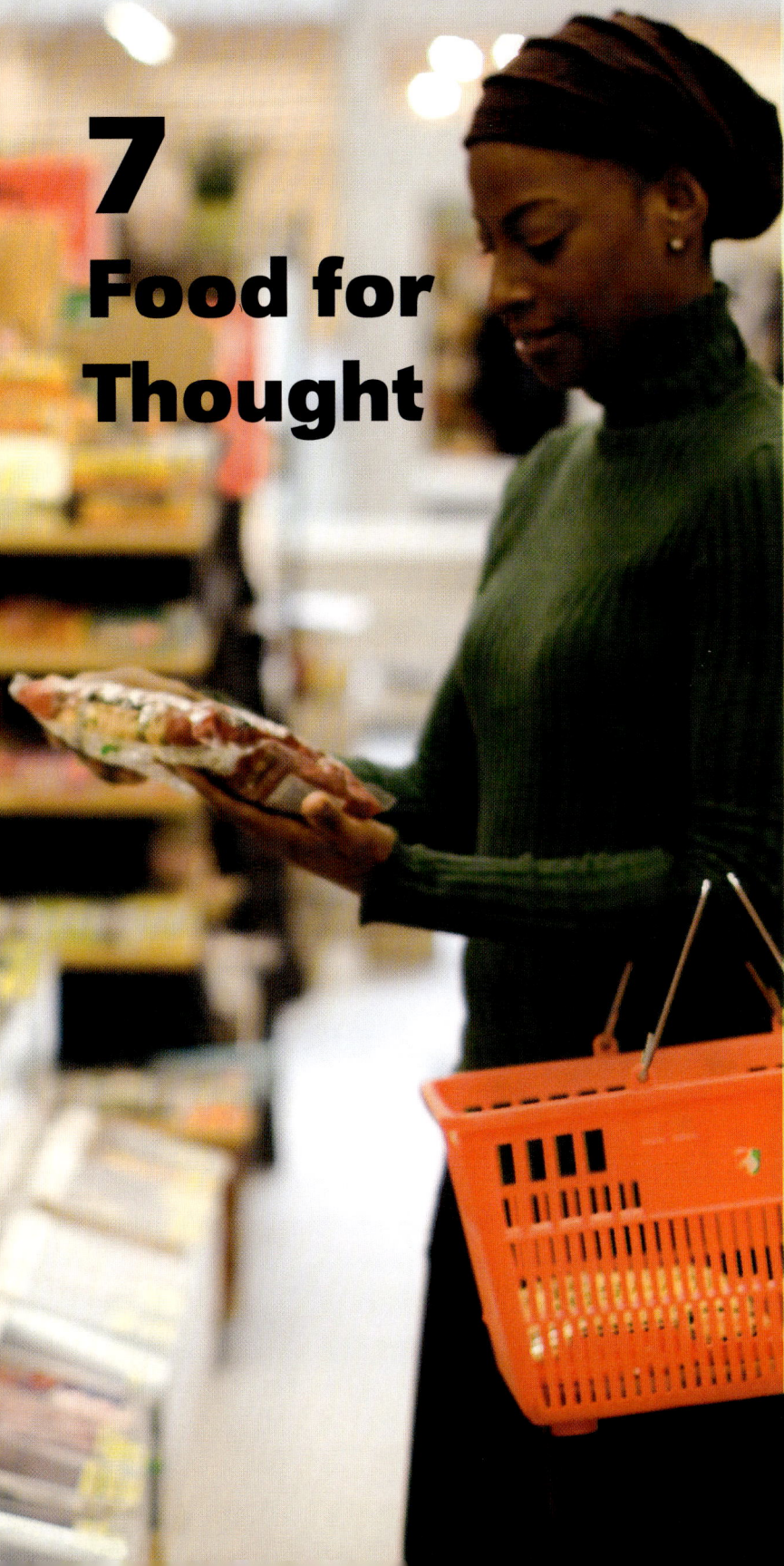

Take a look at your food choices. Are you eating a wide variety of foods? Are most of these foods whole grains, fruits, nuts, and vegetables? They should be. If not, think about how you can swap one food for another. For example, if you start every day with a sugar doughnut, switch to oatmeal or whole-wheat toast. If you still want that doughnut (and you probably will), think of it as a treat and have it only on special occasions.

Now take a look at the variety of foods in your diet. Do you eat mainly from the meat category? Do you eat only vegetables? As mentioned several times in this book, it is important to have variety in your diet. If you're vegetarian, it's important that you find a source of adequate iron and protein. If you're only eating red meat, you could be on your way to high cholesterol and high blood pressure, among other health conditions. Red meat isn't completely bad, but it should be eaten in moderation. Try having salmon or another fatty fish at least once a week.

How much you eat is important no matter what you eat. According to most nutrition experts, portion size in

Think about what you eat. Make a habit of reading package labels. The best time to make decisions about nutrition is not when you're hungry—so plan ahead.

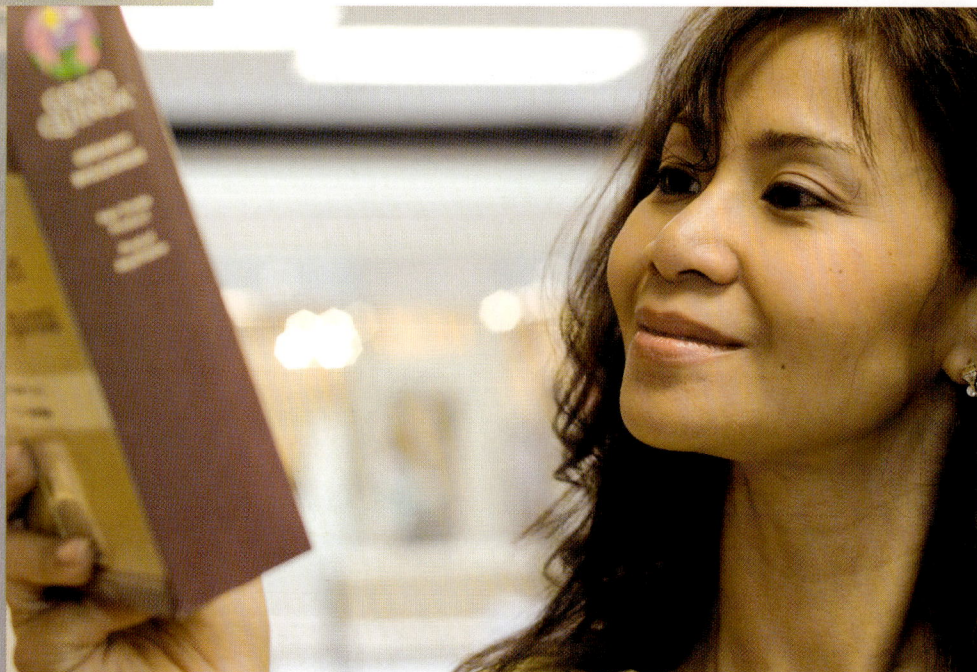

the United States is way out of control. Many people have only a vague idea what a serving size is. For example, what is a small baked potato? It's about the size of your fist—or a computer mouse.

How to Eat

"How to eat" might seem pretty obvious. If you can read this book, you certainly know how to eat. But do you really?

Many of us are so busy that we eat very quickly. You've barely sat down (if you've bothered to do that) before your meal is over. Try something different: dine instead of "gobble." Sit down, take your time, put your eating utensil down between bites, chew, taste the food. Make it an experience. Enjoy the food. If you're with someone, talk to them. If not, consider reading a book while you eat.

If you're out with friends and tempted to go to a drive-through, suggest that you go inside and sit at a table. Or take the food to a park and have a picnic.

So does it really make a difference *how* you eat? Yes. By turning mealtime into an experience instead of a **pit stop**, you have slowed down your eating. This gives your body time to get full, and you won't eat as much.

What About Physical Activity?

Though there is still a lot to discover about nutrition and health, one thing is clear: physical activity goes hand in hand with good nutrition. That doesn't mean everyone needs to be an athletic; they just need to be active.

Getting more activity into your life doesn't mean you need to join an organized sport. Take the stairs instead of the lift, park further away from your destination and walk,

---

Ask the Doctor

Q: I am trying to be a vegetarian, but my mother keeps telling me it's not healthy. I'm willing to compromise for now and just eat fish. Can I tell her that it's okay to eat only fish—no meat?

Yes, but remember to have a variety of fish in your diet. Don't eat just salmon or just tuna. You can also eat eggs, milk, cheese, nuts, beans, and soy products. Tell your mother that these are also good sources of protein. And be sure to include a variety of vegetables and whole-grain foods in your diet as well. People who are vegetarians can have healthy nutrition—but like everyone, you need to be careful what you eat and be sure you're getting all the nutrients you need.

play a pickup game of football with your friends, get off the bus a couple stops earlier than usual, go for a bicycle ride, walk to school. Keep in mind, though, that if it's been a while since you've exercised or you have extra weight, start slowly and build up. For example, if you need to go up four flights of stairs, start by going up one or two and take the elevator the rest of the way. You'll still get some of the benefits, but you won't be **overtaxed** and discouraged.

The Special Issue of Obesity

Obesity, and with it diabetes, heart disease and other weight-related conditions, is becoming a worldwide issue. In most cases, weight loss can be achieved through a modified diet and increased activity. "Fad" diets might work in the short term, but it's been proven time and again that the results don't last. Individuals who need to

Your relationship with food shapes who you are emotionally, physically, and mentally.

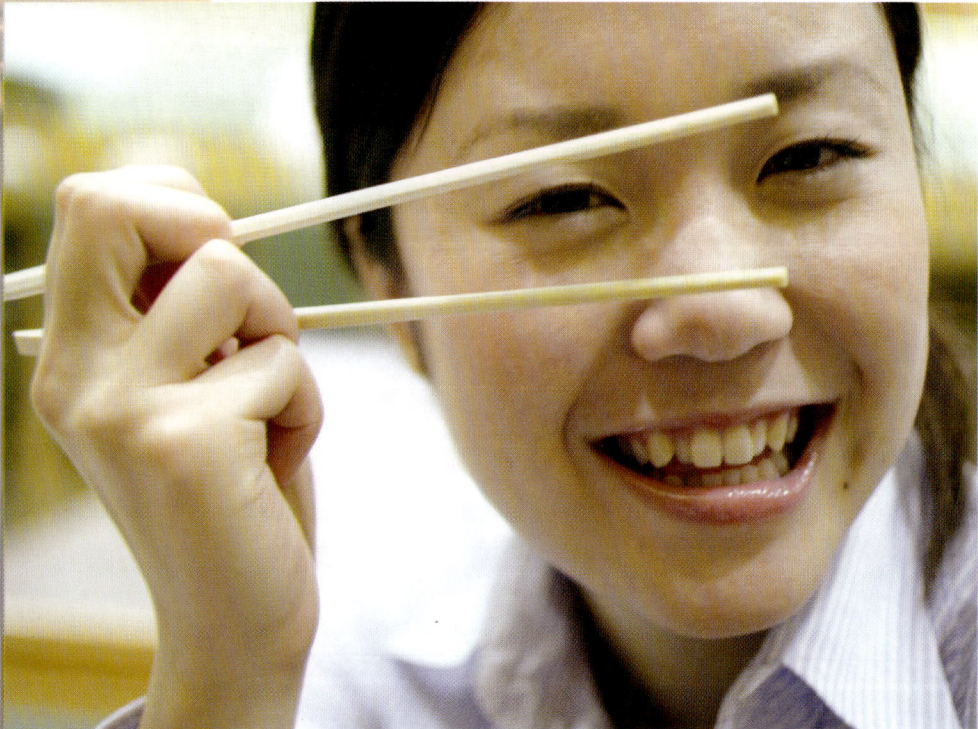

lose weight still need to eat a healthy diet from all of the food groups.

Remember, if you need to lose weight, do it because it will make you healthier. Weight-loss programs begun at someone else's urging or to fit into a special outfit usually don't work. And as with the fad diets, any weight lost usually comes back—and then some.

Your Relationship with Food

When you were younger, you probably didn't have all that much control over what you ate. The grownups in your life made the decisions about what went on the table—and in your mouth. But as you grow older, more and more of the responsibility for taking care of yourself physically will be all yours. This includes deciding what you eat.

None of us can completely control the quality of our nutrition. It depends on factors outside our control, like where we live, how much money we have, and our cultural traditions. But within that framework, it's up to you: are you going to make nutrition a priority in your life? Your body will thank you if you do.

Did You Know?

Most dietary guidelines list three ounces as the serving size for fish. That's about the size of a checkbook.

FIVE NUTRITION MYTHS

1. Vegetarian diets are healthier.

Fact: *Vegetarian diets can be very healthy—but not if your vegetarian diet means French fries, cookies, and chips! If you want to stop eating meat and fish, you make sure you include other foods that will give you the protein and vitamins and minerals, such as iron and zinc, that you would normally get from meat.*

2. Dairy products make you fat.

Fact: *Eating more than our bodies need means we put on weight (no matter what we eat). So to keep a healthy weight it's important to follow a balanced diet and keep physically active. The fat content of dairy products varies a lot, and much of this fat is saturated fat, which can raise cholesterol and is linked to heart disease. So although eating dairy products won't make you fat, some are high in saturated fat and so you should only eat small amounts, or eat them less often. Or you could choose reduced-fat versions instead. Dairy products such as milk, cheese and yoghurt are an important part of a healthy balanced diet because they are great sources of protein and vitamins A, B12, and D. They're also an important source of calcium, which helps to keep our bones strong. This is important for everyone but especially if you're into sports. The calcium in dairy foods is easy for the body to absorb. Cutting out dairy products can be bad for your health because you could be missing out on these nutrients. Go for semi-skimmed or skimmed milk and low-fat yoghurts. These contain at least the same amount of protein, B vitamins, calcium, magnesium, phosphorus, potassium, and zinc as full-fat versions, but they contain less saturated fat.*

3. If you take a vitamin supplement in the morning you don't need to worry about what you eat the rest of the day.
Fact: *Although vitamin supplements may provide all the vitamins you need each day, there are lots of other important nutrients they don't provide. So it's still important to choose a healthy balanced diet. Remember, vitamin supplements are no substitute for a healthy diet.*

4. Diet drinks don't damage your teeth.
Fact: *Even diet drinks can damage your teeth, if you drink too many of them. They are often acidic, and this means they can damage the enamel that protects our teeth. Water or milk are the best things to drink if you want to look after your teeth. If you decide to drink diet drinks, do your teeth a favor and drink them only at mealtimes. Diet versions of fizzy drinks also contain very few nutrients, so milk or water are much healthier choices.*

5. Skipping meals is a good way to lose weight.
Fact: *Skipping meals is not a good way to lose weight. Eating three small meals a day and a couple of healthy snacks (such as a piece of fruit, a low-fat yoghurt, or a bowl of cereal) in between is a much better way to control your calories. And getting active is the best way to make sure you burn off as much as you take in.*

(Source: UK Food Standards Agency, www.eatwell.gov.uk)

STRAIGHT FROM THE SOURCE

(From the WHO, Chinese Ministry of Health (MoH) and Beijing Food Safety Administration (BFA) document, WHO and China Call for Safer Food, Healthier Diets and Regular Exercise to Welcome 2008 Olympic Games In China)

The Olympics and Nutrition

As the Olympic Games express the true excellence of fitness and health, the launch of 'The 3 Fives' in connection with the Beijing Olympics becomes part of the Olympics tradition with national and international implications for public health.

Five Keys to Safer Food:

• Food handlers should keep hands, surfaces and equipment clean when handling food;

• Separate raw and cooked food, especially meat, poultry and seafood;

• Cook food thoroughly to kill bacteria;

• Keep food at safe temperatures to avoid bacterial growth;

• Use safe water and raw materials to avoid bacteria and toxic chemicals.

Five Keys to a Healthy Diet:

• Exclusive breast-feeding for the first 6 months of life;

• People should eat a variety of foods to assure an adequate and balanced diet;

• This includes plenty of fruits and vegetables;

• Moderate intake of fats and oils;

• Reduced intake of salt and sugars.

Five Keys to Appropriate Physical Activity:

- Everybody is encouraged to increase their levels of physical activity and reduce sedentary activities;

- Be physically active every day in as many ways as you can;

- Do at least 30 minutes of moderate-intensity physical activity on 5 or more days each week;

- If you can, enjoy some regular vigorous-intensity physical activity for extra health and fitness benefits;

School-aged children in particular should engage in at least 60 minutes of moderate to vigorous-intensity physical activity each day.

What Do You Think?

- What are the 3 Fives?

- Why do WHO, MoH and the BFA feel these are important to promote at this time? Do you agree?

- How can you help promote the 3 Fives in your own community?

Find Out More

Think more about your relationship with food while checking out these Web sites:

Eatwell, UK Food Standards Agency
www.eatwell.gov.uk/agesandstages/teens/

Meals Matter
www.mealsmatter.org/topics/article.aspx?articleID=52

Teens and Nutrition
www.ext.colostate.edu/pubs/COLUMNCC/cc970626.html

For More Information on Nutrition

Books

Blake, Joan Salge. *Nutrition and You.* San Francisco, Calif.: Benjamin Cummings, 2007.

DK Publishing. *Food.* New York: DK, 2005.

Esherick, Joan. *Diet and Your Emotions: The Comfort Food Falsehood.* Broomall, Pa.: Mason Crest, 2005.

Flynn, Noa. *When Food Is an Enemy: Youth with Eating Disorders.* Broomall, Pa.: Mason Crest, 2008.

Gay, Kathlyn. *Am I Fat? The Obesity Issue for Teens.* Berkeley Heights, N.J.: Enslow, 2006.

Hunnicut, Susan C. *World Hunger.* Farmington Hills, Mich.: Greenhaven, 2006.

Libal, Autumn. *The Importance of Physical Activity and Exercise: The Fitness Factor.* Broomall, Pa.: Mason Crest, 2005.

Nestle, Marion. *Food Politics.* Los Angeles: University of California Press, 2007.

———. *Safer Food.* Los Angeles: University of California Press, 2004.

Orr, Tamra B. *When the Mirror Lies: Anorexia, Bulimia, and Other Eating Disorders.* New York: Franklin Watts, 2006.

Schlosser, Eric and Charles Wilson. *Chew on This: Everything You Don't Want to Know About Fast Food.* New York: Houghton Mifflin, 2006.

Shanley, Ellen, and Colleen Thompson. *Fueling the Teen Machine*. Palo Alto, Calif.: Bull Publishing, 2001.

Thompson, Janice and Melinda Manore. *Food for Life*. San Francisco, Calif.: Benjamin Cummings, 2006.

Turck, Mary. *Food and Emotions*. Mankato, Minn.: Life-Matters, 2001.

Young, Liz. *World Hunger*. Philadelphia, Pa.: Routledge, 2007.

Web Sites

NRG: Powered by Choice
www.poweredbychoice.org/about/index.php

Nutrition Data
www.nutritiondata.com

Nutrition Explorations
www.nutritionexplorations.org

One
www.one.org

United Nations World Food Program
www.wfp.org/

USDA Food and Nutrition Information Center
fnic.nal.usda.gov/nal_display/index.php?info_center=4&tax_level=1

U.S. Federal Guide to Nutrition
www.nutrition.gov

U.S. My Pyramid
www.mypyramid.gov

World Health Organization
www.who.org

World Hunger: Facts, Figures, and Statistics
library.thinkquest.org/C002291/high/present/stats.htm

World Hunger Notes
www.worldhunger.org/articles/Learn/
world%20hunger%20facts%202002.ht

Glossary of Nutrition-Related Terms

As you read about nutrition and nutrition-related issues, you'll probably come across terms you may not completely understand, even though they may sound familiar. This glossary will help you better understand many of the topics that have to do with nutrition. You may also find it useful for helping you to understand the ingredients listed on food labels.

additives (food additives)
Any natural or synthetic material, other than the basic raw ingredients, used in a food item to enhance the final product. Any substance that may affect the characteristics of any food, including those used in the production, processing, treatment, packaging, transportation, or storage of food.

algin
A chemical which comes from algae and is used in puddings, milk shakes, and ice cream to make these foods creamier and thicker and to extend shelf life.

alitame
A sweetener made from amino that offers a taste that is 2000 times sweeter than that of sucrose and can be used in a wide variety of products including beverages, table-top sweeteners, frozen desserts, and baked goods. Since alitame is such an intense sweetener, it is used at very low levels and contributes very few calories. The U.S. FDA is currently considering a petition to approve its use in the United States food supply. So far, alitame has been approved for use in all food and beverage products in Australia, Mexico and New Zealand.

allergen
A food allergen is the part of a food that stimulates the immune system of individuals who are allergic to a specific food. A single food can contain multiple food allergens. Carbohydrates and fats are never allergens, but certain proteins are.

allergy

A food allergy is any adverse reaction to an otherwise harmless food or food component that involves the body's immune system.

alpha carotene

A chemical found in carrots that provides the health benefit of neutralizing free radicals that may cause damage to cells that could lead to cancer.

amino acids

Amino acids function as the building blocks of proteins. They are classified as essential and nonessential and conditionally essential. Essential amino acids cannot be made by the body and must be supplied as part of the diet. Nonessential amino acids can be synthesized by the body in adequate amounts.

anemia

Anemia is a condition in which there are not enough healthy red blood cells, which affects the exchange of oxygen and carbon dioxide between the blood and the body's other cells. Most anemias are caused by a lack of nutrients, but a chronic disease or drugs can cause anemia as well.

anorexia nervosa

An eating disorder that includes weight loss; an intense fear of weight gain or becoming fat, despite the individual's being underweight status; an inaccurate self-awareness body weight or shape; and in females, the absence of at least three consecutive menstrual cycles that would otherwise be expected to occur.

anticarcinogens

Substances that help prevent cancers from forming. More than 600 chemicals are said to be anticancer agents, including natural chemicals in garlic, broccoli, cabbage, and green tea.

antioxidants
Antioxidants may help to maintain overall health. Studies show that antioxidants may be able to help fight off toxic oxygen molecules (often called "**free radicals**"), a byproduct of metabolism that can damage cells.

ascorbic acid
Also known as vitamin C, it is essential for the development and maintenance of connective tissue. Vitamin C speeds the production of new cells in wound healing and it is an antioxidant that keeps free radicals from hooking up with other molecules to form damaging compounds that might attack tissue. Vitamin C protects the immune system, helps fight off infections, reduces the severity of allergic reactions, and plays a role in the synthesis of hormones and other body chemicals. Green peppers, broccoli, citrus fruits, tomatoes, strawberries, and other fresh fruits and vegetables are good sources of vitamin C.

aspartame
A low calorie sweetener used in a variety of foods and beverages and as a tabletop sweetener. It is about 200 times sweeter than sugar.

beta glucan
A soluble fiber in oats which provides the health benefit of reducing the risk of cardiovascular disease by decreasing circulating blood cholesterol.

BHA
Butylated hydroxyanisole, a chemical compound used to preserve foods by preventing rancidity. BHA is found in foods high in fats and oils; also in meats, cereals, baked goods, beer, and snack foods.

BHT
Butylated hydroxytoluene, a chemical compound used to keep food from changing flavor, odor, and/or color. It is added to foods high in fats and oils and cereals.

BMI
Body Mass Index is an index of a person's weight in relation to height, determined by dividing weight (in kilograms) by the square of the height (in meters).

BMR
Basal Metabolic Rate is the rate of energy used for metabolism when the body is at complete rest.

bulimia nervosa
An eating disorder characterized by rapid consumption of a large amount of food in a short period of time. There are two forms of the condition: purging and non-purging. People with the first type regularly engages in purging through self-induced vomiting or the use of laxatives or diuretics. The non-purging type controls weight through strict dieting, fasting, or excessive exercise.

caffeine
A natural stimulant found in many foods and beverages, including coffee, tea, cola drinks, and chocolate.

calcium
A mineral that you need for strong bones and teeth. Calcium is found in dairy products (like milk and cheese) and also in dried beans and dark green vegetables (like spinach).

calorie
A unit of measure, sometimes referred to as a kilocalorie. Calories measure the amount of energy your body can get from a food. Calories are found in fats, carbohydrates, proteins, and alcohol.

carbohydrates
Sugars and starches are the main forms of carbohydrates. Sugars are simple carbohydrates and starches, such as breads, cereals and pasta, are complex carbohydrates. Each gram of carbohydrate provides four calories of energy.

carcinogens
Substances that cause cancer within the body.

carotene
Also known as beta-carotene, a yellow pigment (found in food) that may be converted into Vitamin A in the body.

catechins
A chemical found in tea which provides the health benefits of neutralizing free radicals and possibly reducing the risk of cancer.

cholesterol
Cholesterol is a soft, waxy substance found among the lipids (fats) in the bloodstream and in all your body's cells. It is used to form cell membranes, some hormones, and other needed tissues. However, a high level of cholesterol in the blood is a major risk factor for coronary heart disease.

coronary heart disease
Conditions related to the heart and blood vessels leading to and from the heart. Most common symptoms are chest pains, heart attacks, stroke, and high blood pressure.

cyclamate
A sweetener that is 30 times sweeter than sucrose and calorie free. It is approved for tabletop use in Canada and more than 50 countries in Europe, Asia, South America and Africa. Since 1970, however, the use of cyclamate has been banned in the United States on the basis of a study that suggested that cyclamates may be related to the development of bladder tumors in rats.

diabetes
A group of medical disorders characterized by high blood sugar levels. Normally when people eat, food is digested and much of it is converted to glucose—a simple sugar— which the body uses for energy. The blood carries the glu-

cose to cells where it is absorbed with the help of the hormone insulin. For people with diabetes, however, the body does not make enough insulin, or cannot properly use the insulin it does make. Without insulin, glucose accumulates in the blood rather than moving into the cells. High blood sugar levels result.

diet
What you eat every day.

digestion
The process where your body breaks down food into smaller parts it can use.

eating disorders
Psychological conditions where a person's relationship with food becomes unhealthy. Bulimia and anorexia are both examples.

energy
The body's capacity for doing work. Food gives us the energy we need to live, work, and play.

enriched
Indicates that more of the food's natural nutrients have been added during processing. This is often done to replace nutrients that may have been lost through handling.

fat
These are concentrated sources of energy. Every gram of fat provides nine calories.

fat replacers
Fat replacers are developed to duplicate the taste and texture of fat, but contain fewer calories per gram than fat.

fiber
Part of plants which the body cannot digest, it helps your digestive system and intestines keep working well.

5 A Day

The dietary recommendation to consume five servings of fruits and vegetables every day.

flavanones

A chemical found in citrus fruits that provides the health benefits of neutralizing **free radicals** and possibly reducing the risk of cancer.

flavones

A chemical found in various fruits and vegetables that provides the health benefits of neutralizing **free radicals** and possibly reducing the risk of cancer.

folic acid

Chemicals that help with the digestion of protein. Good dietary sources of folate include leafy, dark green vegetables, legumes, citrus fruits and juices, peanuts, whole grains, and fortified breakfast cereals. Recent studies show that if all women of childbearing age consumed sufficient folic acid (either through diet or supplements), 50 to 70 percent of birth defects of the brain and spinal cord could be prevented.

food intolerance

A general term for any adverse reaction to a food or food component that does not involve the body's immune system.

food preservatives

Preservatives prevent spoilage either by slowing the growth of organisms that live on food or by protecting the food from oxygen.

fortified

When nutrients not naturally found in that particular food have been added during processing to enhance nutrition.

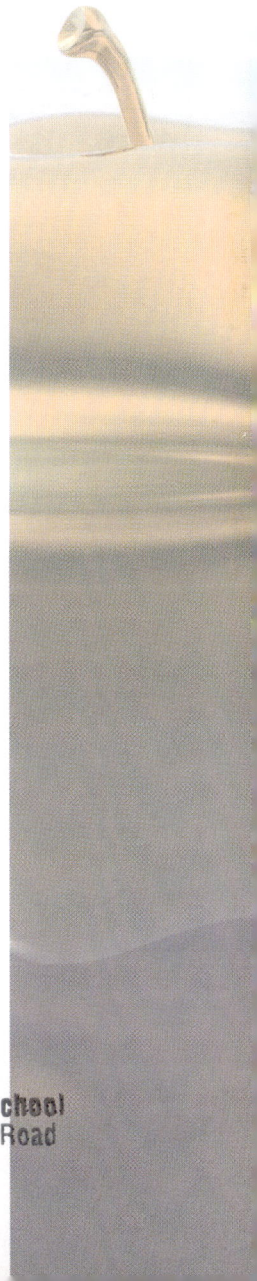

Garibaldi Secondary School
24789 Dewdney Trunk Road
Maple Ridge, B.C.
V4R 1X2

free radicals
Chemicals released when unsaturated fatty acids decompose and which may contribute to cancer growth.

fructose
Fructose is a sugar found naturally in fruits; it is also a component of high fructose corn syrup.

glucose
A natural sugar that comes from grape juice, honey, and certain vegetables, among other things.

glycerin
A syrupy type of alcohol derived from sugar that is used in food flavorings to maintain desired food consistency.

glycerol
A colorless, odorless, syrupy liquid that is obtained from fats and oils and used to retain moisture and add sweetness to foods.

grains
The seeds or fruits of various food plants, including cereal grasses, such as wheat, corn, oats, barley, rye, and rice. Grain foods include foods such as bread, cereals, rice, and pasta.

guar gum
A substance made from the seeds of the guar plant that acts as a stabilizer in foods. Is found as a food additive in cheese, ice cream, and dressings.

high fructose corn syrup
A sweet syrup that generally contains 42 percent, 55 percent or 90 percent fructose, which is used in products such as soft drinks or cake mixes.

iron
A mineral that is an important part of hemoglobin, your blood's oxygen-carrying molecule within red blood cells.

Iron also helps your body resist infection and use energy from food.

lactose intolerance
Lactose intolerance is an inherited inability to properly digest dairy products. Symptoms of lactose intolerance, including abdominal cramps, gas, and diarrhea, can increase with age.

lecithin
A byproduct of soybean oil, it is also found in eggs, red meats, spinach, and nuts. It is used in some commercial foods as a lubricant, and it promotes "good" cholesterol levels.

lipids
Chemicals that include fats and oils.

lycopene
The chemical that gives tomatoes and some other fruits and vegetables their red color. It is a good antioxidant that helps keep cells healthy.

malnutrition
Poor nutrition resulting in tiredness, illness, lack of ability to fight infection, and finally muscle wasting in the latter stages.

metabolism
The chemical reactions that go on in living cells by which energy is produced for use by the cells.

MSG (monosodium glutamate)
A flavoring found in many packaged foods and in Chinese foods. In the early part of the century, MSG was extracted from seaweed and other plant sources. Today, MSG is produced in many countries around the world through a fermentation process of molasses from sugar cane or sugar beets, as well as starch and corn sugar.

nitrite

Nitrite is a food additive that has been used for centuries to preserve meats, fish and poultry. It also contributes to the characteristic flavor, color, and texture of processed meats such as hot dogs.

nutrients

Components in food that our bodies use for survival, including fats, carbohydrates, protein, vitamins, and minerals.

nutrient density

Nutrient-dense foods are those that provide substantial amounts of vitamins and minerals and relatively fewer calories. The opposite of nutrient dense is calorie dense, foods that mainly supply calories and relatively few nutrients.

obesity

A chronic disease characterized by excessively high body fat in relation to lean body tissue.

omega 3 fatty acids

A type of fatty acid found in fish and marine oils that provide the health benefits of reduced risk of cardiovascular disease and improved mental and visual function.

organic

Agricultural products that are grown using cultural, biological, and mechanical methods rather than chemicals to control pests, improve soil quality, and enhance processing.

overweight

An excess of body fat.

phytochemicals

Chemicals found in plants and vegetables, some of which have been found to help protect against some cancers, heart disease, and other chronic health conditions.

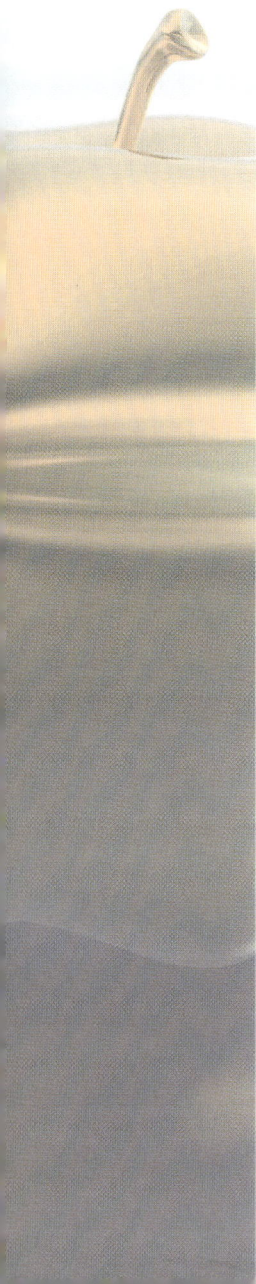

poultry
Meat that comes from birds, like chickens, ducks, geese, and turkeys.

protein
Building blocks that our body uses, which are made up of chains of amino acids. Body tissues, like our skin, hair, and muscles, are built mostly of protein. Protein is also needed for our bodies' growth and repair.

refined
Refers to the fine grinding and sifting of cereal grains to produce white flour.

saccharin
Saccharin is the oldest of the "artificial" sweeteners. It is 300 times sweeter than sucrose, heat stable, and does not promote dental cavities. Saccharin has a long shelf life, but a slightly bitter aftertaste. It is not metabolized in the human digestive system, is excreted rapidly in the urine, and does not accumulate in body.

saturated fat
Fatty acids that have all the hydrogen they can hold on their chemical chains. They mainly come from animal foods and tend to deposit in blood vessels, blocking blood flow.

sodium (Na)
Part of the chemical that makes up table salt. This mineral is used for cellular fluid balance,and muscle retractions.

sodium nitrite
A salt used in smoked or cured fish and in meat curing preparation. It acts as a preservative and color fixative. Can combine with chemicals in the stomach to form a carcinogenic substance.

soluble fiber
A type of dietary fiber found in psyllium, cereals, oatmeal, apples, citrus fruits, beans, and other foods that reduces

high blood cholesterol levels, which in turn decreases the risk of cardiovascular disease.

soy protein
The protein found in soybeans and soy-based foods, which when consumed at the level of 25 grams per day may reduce the risk of heart disease.

starch
A complex carbohydrate that our bodies break down and uses for energy.

sugar
A simple carbohydrate that our bodies break down and uses for energy.

sulfites
Sulfiting agents are sometimes used to preserve the color of foods such as dried fruits and vegetable, and to inhibit the growth of microorganisms in fermented foods such as wine. Sulfites are safe for most people. A small segment of the population, however, has been found to develop shortness of breath or fatal shock shortly after exposure to these preservatives. Sulfites can provoke severe asthma attacks in sulfite sensitive asthmatics. For that reason, in 1986 the U.S. FDA banned the use of sulfites on fresh fruits and vegetables (except potatoes) intended to be sold or served raw to consumers. Sulfites added to all packaged and processed foods must be listed on the product label.

trans fats
Trans fats occur naturally in many meats, butter, and milk, as well as in commercially prepared margarines and solid cooking fats. The main sources of trans fats in people's diet today are margarine, shortening, commercial frying fats, and high-fat baked goods. Trans fats can raise "bad" cholesterol and lower "good" cholesterol.

triglycerides

The scientific name for the common form of fat, found in both the body and in foods. Most body fat is stored in the form of triglycerides.

unsaturated fat

This type of fat has been found to be better for health and may protect against heart disease. It is mainly found in vegetables and fish.

vegetarian

A person whose diet excludes some or all protein from animal sources. Semi-vegetarians will not eat red meat but will eat fish and poultry. Lacto-ovo vegetarians eat no meats but will eat dairy products and eggs. Lacto vegetarians eat no meat, only dairy products. Vegans are strict vegetarians, and eat no foods from animals at all, only from plant sources.

vitamins

A group of nutrients that our bodies need to grow and function well. Some important vitamins that we need are B vitamins, and vitamin A, C, D, E and K.

whole grain

A term that applies to grains in which the outer layer, where the B vitamins and minerals are concentrated, is not removed during processing.

Bibliography

Asfaw, Abay. "Obesity and Chronic Diseases: Not Limited to the Affluent." International Food Policy Research Institute. http://www.ifpri.org/pubs/newsletters/IFPRI-Forum/200612/if17.

Britten, Patricia, Kristin Marcoe, Sedigheh Yamini, and Carole Davis. "Development of Food Intake Patterns for the MyPyramid Food Guidance System." *J. Nutrition Education and Behavior* vol. 38 (December 2006): S78–S92.

Damsgaard, C. T., L. Lauritzen, and T. M. Kjaer. "Fish Oil Supplementation Modulates Immune Function in Healthy Infants." *J. Nutrition* vol. 137 (April 2007): 1031–1036.

"Diet and Nutrition." Time. http://www.time.com/time/archive/collections/0,21428,c_diet_and_nutrition,00.shtml.

Green, K. N., H. Martinez-Coria, and H. Khashwji. "Dietary docosahexaenoic acid and docosapentaenoic acid ameliorate amyloid-beta and tau pathology via a mechanism involving presenilin 1 levels." *J. Neuroscience* vol. 27 (April 2007): 4385–4395.

"Eat the Basic 7 Every Day." http://digital.library.unt.edu/permalink/meta-dc-619:1.

Farney, Teresa J. "Good Mood Food: Researchers Find Links Between Nutrition and the Brain Chemicals Governing Our Inner World." *The Gazette*, September 18, 2002.

International Food Information Council. "Child & Adolescent Nutrition, Health & Physical Activity." http://ific.org/nutrition/kids/index.cfm?renderforprint=1.

Ryan, Monique. *Sports Nutrition for Endurance Athletes.* Boulder, Col.: VeloPress, 2007.

"Sports Nutrition: Dietary Needs." http://www.drug-freesport.com/choices/nutrition/dietary.html.

Squires, Sally. "Pyramid Schemes: Taking a Global Perspective on Nutrition." *Washington Post*, July 4, 2000.

Stang, J., and M. Story (eds.). *Guidelines for Adolescent Nutrition Services.* Minneapolis: University of Minnesota, 2005.

WHO. FAO/WHO Launch Expert Report on Diet, Nutrition, and Prevention of Chronic Diseases." 2003. http://www.who.int/mediacentre/news/releases/2003/pr32/en.

Willett, Walter C., and P. J. Skettett. *Eat, Drink, and Be Healthy: The Harvard Medical School Guide to Healthy Eating.* New York: Free Press, 2005.

Index

Picture Credits

Dreamstime
   Jahoo: p. 10

Learning Radiology
   p. 71

Health Canada
   p. 23

University of Bath
   p. 50

Jupiter Images
   pp. 9, 12, 14, 17, 19,
28–29, 30, 32, 41–42, 45,
48–49, 58–60, 63, 68–70,
74, 82–84, 86

USDA
   p. 21

To the best knowledge of the publisher, all other images are in the public domain. If any image has been inadvertently uncredited, please notify Harding House Publishing Service, Vestal, New York 13850, so that rectification can be made for future printings.

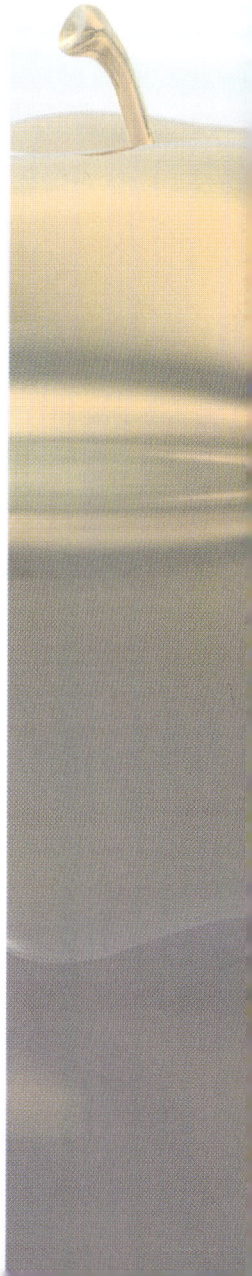

About the Author

Ida Walker is a freelance author and editor living in upstate New York. She has written many books for middle-grade and young-adult readers. She is also the publisher of Tummy Growl, an ezine about food and cooking.

About the Consultant

Elise DeVore Berlan, MD, MPH, FAAP, is a faculty member of the Division of Adolescent Health at Nationwide Children's Hospital and an Assistant Professor of Clinical Pediatrics at The Ohio State University College of Medicine. She completed her Fellowship in Adolescent Medicine at Children's Hospital Boston and obtained a Master's Degree in Public Health at the Harvard School of Public Health. Dr. Berlan completed her residency in pediatrics at the Children's Hospital of Philadelphia, where she also served an additional year as Chief Resident. She received her medical degree from the University of Iowa College of Medicine. Dr. Berlan is board certified in Pediatrics and board eligible in Adolescent Medicine. She provides primary care and consultative services in the area of Young Women's Health, including gynecological problems, concerns about puberty, reproductive health services, and reproductive endocrine disorders.

Peter Vash, M.D., is a Professor of Medicine at UCLA Medical Center. He is a Fellow of the American Association of Clinical Endocrinologists and a board-certified internist specializing in metabolism and obesity. He is also the author of *The Fat to Muscle Diet*, *The Dieter's Dictionary*, and *A Matter of Fat*.

Garibaldi Secondary School
24789 Dewdney Trunk Road
Maple Ridge, B.C.
V4R 1X2